Paul Zoll MD

The Pioneer Whose Discoveries Prevent Sudden Death

Paul Zoll MD
The Pioneer Whose Discoveries Prevent Sudden Death

By Stafford I. Cohen

Copyright © 2014 by Stafford I. Cohen

ISBN: 978-0-9838131-6-3 (hardcover)
ISBN: 978-0-9838131-7-0 (paperback)

Library of Congress Control Number: 2014938470

Free People Publishing
Salem, N.H.

Cover design by Josh Hartley

Text layout and design by
Zynt Author Services

Cover photo courtesy of Ruth and David Freiman Archives
at Beth Israel Deaconess Medical Center

Printed in the United States of America

This book is dedicated to Deborah, my wife of 53 years, who has helped me chase and catch my dreams.

It is also dedicated to the preservationists of medical history. In their midst is an outstanding group of individuals who culled through their collective memories to contribute to this biography. Most, but not all, are mentioned in the End Notes.

CONTENTS

Photos, Tables and Diagrams

ACKNOWLEDGMENTS

During my 40 year practice of cardiology, generous individuals and the Simons Foundation made financial contributions to a fund designated to help my commitment to research and teaching. This book would not have been possible without their support and that of others who offered other forms of aid. I was encouraged by Mark Josephson M.D., Chief of Cardiovascular Medicine at Beth Israel Deaconess Medical Center, and by Steven Korn, former Futura Publishing co-founder and current President of Science International Corporation. Steven knew most of the contemporary pioneers in the field of electrocardiac therapy. He told me that *this is a book that must be written.*

Elizabeth Prendergast was of enormous assistance in searching the internet to locate persons of interest as well as providing transcription services. Trudy Schrandt also helped with transcriptions. Special thanks to Betsy Bogdansky of the Heart Rhythm Foundation for making NASPE/ HEART RHYTHM SOCIETY Rhythm in Time interviews available for my review.

My principal goal was to write a scholarly work about Paul Zoll and his era of rapid advance in electrocardiac therapy. After completing the research and a draft of the text, I concluded that the effort should not only add to the body of medical history, but also should be understood by curious or involved laypersons. Jeffrey Zygmont, having that mindset, became my editor and requested that I describe concepts, terms and technology in easily understandable, layman's language. Mr. Zygmont has my deepest gratitude for helping craft this effort.

Every attempt has been made to trace the copyright holders of texts and images reproduced here. Should copyright holders make themselves known after publication, due acknowledgment will gladly be made.

FORWARD

By Historian of Medicine Kirk Jeffrey

There is a long history of physicians writing about medical advances in their special fields. In the electrical treatment of cardiac arrhythmias, the papers of David C. Schechter, published in the New York State Journal of Medicine in 1971-72 and gathered in a reprint edition entitled *Exploring the Origins of Electrical Cardiac Stimulation* (Minneapolis: Medtronic, 1983), are outstanding examples. Schechter seemed to have read every scientific paper in every European language on electricity in medicine going back to the mid-18th century.

But Stafford Cohen's new biography of Paul M. Zoll is something different. Dr. Cohen, a cardiologist, knew Zoll as a mentor, colleague, and friend. He has not only re-read Zoll's scientific publications but interviewed the great scientist's colleagues, patients, family, and even neighbors. He gives the reader a sense of Zoll as a man – a man groping with new ideas and recalcitrant technologies, struggling to be understood, confident of the fundamental significance of his work but at times impatient with the ideas of other inventors outside his own group.

During the decade after World War II, Dr. Paul M. Zoll emerged as one of the most prominent innovators in the field of cardiology. It was an era of bold, creative surgeons and cardiologists – Dwight Harken, Alfred Blalock, Helen Taussig, C. Walton Lillehei, Äke Senning – and numerous disruptive transformations in the treatment of heart disease. Innovation in the 1950s occurred in markedly different ways from our own era of gigantic organizations and carefully planned campaigns to resolve scientific uncertainties and develop new treatments.

Today, large companies such as Medtronic and Boston Scientific develop and manufacture medical devices for heart disease. Professional organizations including the American College of Cardiology and the Heart Rhythm Society play an important role in setting standards for clinical care and managing the vast, multi-year clinical trials that are now expected before new medical devices and procedures can be put into widespread use. Crucially, federal agencies oversee the entire field of heart medicine: the National Heart, Lung and Blood Institute within the National Institutes of Health provides much of the funding for research and clinical trials; the Food & Drug Administration (FDA) imposes exacting safety standards for the manufacture and use of medical devices. Since the 1960s, hospital and physician payment has been mediated by the Center for Medicare & Medicaid Services because most people who benefit from modern heart technology are over 65 and thus enrolled in Medicare.

Paul Zoll did not think of himself as an "organization man" and was probably never at ease with the rapid transformations underway in the field of heart medicine. He did much of his formative work before Medicare and before the beginnings of FDA regulation of medical devices. Ironically, his work contributed significantly to defining and ushering in the new era in which we now live, by helping to re-cast cardiologists as people prepared to intervene actively in the heart with the most advanced medical machines and devices. But like all good historical writing, Dr. Cohen's biography of Zoll focuses primarily on describing the conditions and assumptions that prevailed in the past rather than treating the past as interesting simply because it was the precursor to our present.

Readers may be surprised to learn that Zoll maintained a busy private medical practice. His patients often had no knowledge of his work on pace-makers and defibrillators, but liked and trusted him because he had helped a child through an earache or a case of the mumps. World-famous after 1952, Zoll continued to make house calls. When I came to his office in 1990 to conduct an interview (he was 79 at the time), several patients were also waiting to see him.

By the standards of later generations, Zoll's research and development setup was quite small. For most of his years of great achievement, he worked with a handful of associates and trainees at the Beth Israel Hospital in Boston; his laboratory consisted of a single basement room of modest dimensions. Zoll lacked a formal background in electronics but took a summer training course and relied on electrical engineer Alan Belgard, who managed much of the actual product development through his small company, Electrodyne. Zoll and his associates published papers in leading medical journals such as the New England Journal of Medicine, and he made presentations at regional and national medical meetings, but he certainly did not conceive of himself as "marketing" his new medical devices in collaboration with Electrodyne.

More than any other research cardiologist of the 1950s, Paul Zoll had a comprehensive understanding of the new field of cardiac electrostimulation and especially the bottlenecks that scientists and clinicians must avoid if pacemakers were ever to move out of the hospital and into the patient's body. At a conference to discuss chronic cardiac pacing in September 1958, others focused on the problem of designing a pacemaker that would enable the heart to vary its rate based on the patient's level of activity. But the approach posed a complex engineering problem for that era, when transistors were just coming into use in the civilian economy. Most conference participants seemed puzzled and uncertain.

But Zoll firmly dismissed the problem: "One does not have to worry particularly about what the cardiac rate is as long as [it lies] between 60 and 100," he insisted. Coordinating the atria and ventricles was a secondary consideration. "The problem at present is to find something that we can use over a long period of time," hence researchers should be working on batteries, encapsulation for implanted pulse generators, and the design of leads. His strategy proved the correct one, and within two years his group and several others had created fixed-rate ventricular pacemakers that could manage heart block for months at a time from within the patient's body. In the electrical treatment of cardiac arrhythmias, a new era had begun.

Dr. Paul Zoll was a pioneer who led us there, being first to create and successfully employ several devices for cardiac pacing and defibrillation that are the fore bearers of life-saving implements commonly used today. Stafford Cohen's book is the first full-length biography of Dr. Zoll. While it strives for historical accuracy and gives a fair and balanced assessment of Zoll's life and work, its overriding strength is to firmly establish Paul M. Zoll as a compassionate innovator whose treatments and inventions make him a father of modern electrocardiac therapy.

Kirk Jeffrey, Ph.D.
Professor Emeritus of History
Carleton College
Northfield, Minnesota

PROLOGUE

A NOTE FROM THE AUTHOR

Many important leaders who forge momentous change are remembered for what they did, not for the personality and character traits responsible for their success. Paul Maurice Zoll's place in history is assured because of his medical milestones, but who he was and what personal factors contributed to his success have never been deeply explored. Zoll was a very private person and a man of few words. He did not record his personal journey. Nor had anyone else.

After his death in 1999, I realized that I could honor his memory by writing a biography that would present a panoramic view of Paul Zoll, promoting an understanding of the man who introduced the modern methods we use today to treat life-threatening heart rhythms with electric shock.

When I entered medical school in 1957, I met Paul Zoll and became familiar with his closed-chest pacemakers, closed-chest defibrillators and alarmed cardiac monitors – all in clinical use at the time. His implanted long-term pacemakers had been introduced and were saving lives when I completed my studies in 1961. During my post-graduate training at Boston's Beth Israel Hospital, Zoll's success with complex cardiac patients was astonishing. He became my teacher and the mentor who directed me on a career path to cardiology. When my career progressed to the level of staff physician at Beth Israel Hospital, we became colleagues and ultimately office mates. In the common room that we shared, as a practical matter, Paul commandeered the shelf space at the lower levels and gave me access to the higher level shelves because I was a foot taller than he.

We became friends.

Paul Zoll's discoveries were instantly appreciated by cardiologists who worked in critical care because of their high probability of success. As director of an intensive care unit, I applied his science. Dr Zoll's algorithms for managing cardiac arrest worked well, as did the application of his pacemaker and defibrillator machines. His cardiac monitors were a godsend in signaling early warning of impending disaster. I performed temporary pacing, helped install permanent pacemakers, and had an office-based pacemaker follow-up clinic. In time, I became involved in managing the healthcare of each of Paul's close collaborators or members of their families.

My perspective on Paul Zoll comes from those and other experiences throughout my career, experiences that have positioned me in the trenches as well as in an academic ivory tower. I have cared for patients, taught, published original observations, written reviews, edited and contributed chapters to books, reviewed articles for medical journals, and lectured about Dr. Zoll. Through that work, I became committed to telling the Paul Zoll story.

During approximately seven years, I reviewed Dr. Zoll's publications and those of authors who mentioned him. I searched and located his testimony in old court records. Beginning in March 2006, I conducted audio and video interviews with Dr. Zoll's neighbors, friends, co-workers, patients, and other pioneers. I encouraged many to write down anecdotal experiences that I collected, recording the last anecdote in May, 2013. During the intervening years, I gathered information from people scattered in far flung locations throughout the United States and from some foreign countries. Because my interest in Dr. Zoll was well known, some of his acquaintances approached me with important memorabilia. Nearly every person that I asked has cooperated by agreeing to an interview or by contributing an anecdote, a story, or an artifact to the project. As a result, I have a small collection of his letters, early drafts of some manuscripts and some of his early "inventions"—although Dr Zoll did not regard himself as the inventor of his machines. The sum of my research yielded original new information that sharpened the focus and enlarged the field of knowledge about Paul Zoll.

This biography of Paul Zoll documents the high standards and values that permeated his research, his practice of medicine, his advocacy for patients and his resistance to innovations of questionable value. The last was crucial to his success.

I hope that my contribution will add to his legacy.

Stafford I. Cohen, M.D.
May 2014

ONE

THE MOMENT OF DISCOVERY

Paul Zoll was an unlikely hero. He wasn't a stereotypical square-jawed muscleman with super-human powers. In fact, he was just the opposite. He was a member of that small fraction of society labeled "cerebral scientific nerds". He was shy and reclusive, with a slight build, short stature and ears that resembled jug handles. Zoll was more comfortable alone in his research laboratory thinking about complex problems than he was at any social gathering. He brimmed with new ideas and creative insight. His expansive knowledge encompassed an appreciation of prior discoveries and his keen intellect enabled him to improve upon them. Paul Zoll was a physician-cardiologist who always devoted half-time to patients and the rest to exploring solutions for their cardiac problems in his research laboratory. With unyielding determination, Zoll worked tirelessly in pursuit of his scientific goals. Driven by a fundamental desire to promote the well-being of others, he made seminal breakthroughs in confronting the subtleties of an out-of-kilter electrical system embedded within many a human heart. In order to treat life-threatening arrhythmias, his laboratory developed prototype medical devices that are commonplace today, but were a new generation of miraculous life savers when they first appeared in the middle of the 20th Century.

A hero? Yes. Paul saved lives. He saved countless lives and the decedents of the machines that he developed (the cardiac pacemaker, heart rhythm monitor and closed-chest defibrillator) continue to save innumerable lives well after his death in 1999 at the age of 87.

It started with a single life that he could not save. In 1948, Dr. Paul Zoll was caring for a 60-year-old, vibrant woman who suffered fainting spells when her heart intermittently failed to beat. Her cardiac electrical system was flawed. She died after three weeks of intensive treatment. Dr. Zoll, overcome with remorse, vowed to save others with similar problems.

So began his life's crusade.

Zoll recalled his World War II experiences when he had assisted with heart and chest surgery in the European war zone. That work with critically injured soldiers eventually directed him towards an electrical approach to arouse a heart that could, but would not beat. He correctly reasoned that an electric artificial pacemaker might substitute for failed cardiac self-stimulation.

Zoll continued to care for patients while constantly shuttling between bedside and laboratory in search of solutions to their arrhythmias. Working with characteristic determination, Paul took three years to achieve the initial monumental breakthrough that changed his life and redirected the course of medicine.

*On a Saturday morning in his basement research laboratory at Boston's Beth Israel Hospital, he was taking yet another pass at a series of failed experiments to electrically stimulate the heart of a closed-chest, anesthetized dog. Two electrodes were in place. One was positioned in the esophagus behind the heart; the other was opposite the first, attached to a needle placed just below the skin on the front surface of the dog's chest. Both electrodes were connected to a borrowed Grass Company multifunctional physiological stimulator intended for animal research. The stimulator was the size of a small microwave oven. In Zoll's setup, the stimulator, once activated, would send a sequence of electrical impulses through the animal's chest cavity, including the heart within. Undaunted by past failures, his insight and intuition told him that it **should** work. So why not try once again? Hopefully, the heart would beat in response to each artificial stimulus. Every heartbeat was recorded on an old Sandborn electro-cardiograph machine modified by the manufacturer to indirectly visualize heart rhythm on an eerie, rotating fluorescent drum. Each beat was initially brightly inscribed, only to fade and disappear after one revolution.[1]*

Paul must have held his breath when he flicked the switch to the "on" position. What he saw was extraordinary. The stimulator was prompting cardiac contractions. Closed-chest electrical impulses were controlling the dog's heartbeat.

Zoll was elated. He couldn't contain the emotion. Normally quiet and reserved, he rushed out of the lab, collared passing colleagues and escorted them back to witness the historic event.[2]

At that instant, Zoll crossed a threshold to a new era: The Modern Era of Electrocardiac Therapy. Comprehending the impact of that moment, Zoll believed that "the whole problem of cardiac arrest was solved at least in theory."[3] He later claimed to have had a vision of all the advances in the field to come during the next 25 years.[4]

He not only envisioned the future, he created it. Dr. Paul Zoll was at the forefront of most of the important advances that occurred during the next quarter century. His leadership earned him the title "father of modern electrocardiac therapy;" a treatment that remedies life-threatening heart rhythms with cardiac pacemaker or defibrillator-delivered electrical shocks.

This is the story of how he got there and how the machines that this extraordinary man developed helped combat sudden arrhythmic death. Sudden cardiac death is a world-wide problem of enormous magnitude that lesser men than Zoll might have considered insurmountable.

TWO

THE GRIM REAPER UNMASKED

Cardiovascular disease is the leading cause of death in the United States. Half the deaths are sudden. The mid-range estimate of U.S. fatalities is 250,000 to 300,000 each year. That adds up to a life lost every two minutes. When the heart stops pumping blood throughout the body, an oxygen deprived brain results in unconsciousness. Within four minutes there is a rapid transition from the quick to the dead. Sudden cardiac death is a worldwide phenomenon. Everyone on the planet is a potential victim or a possible rescuer. That is why, for centuries, the far flung community of mankind has tried to understand and prevent sudden cardiac death.

The human heart is a sturdy muscle that operates as a magnificent four-chambered mechanical pump that circulates blood throughout the body approximately 70 times each minute, or 36 million strokes each year. All four chambers work as pumps. The two upper chambers, called atria, are smaller. They receive blood as it returns to the heart from the near and far parts of the body and then pump it into the larger chambers beneath them, which are called the ventricles. The right ventricle pumps blood into the lungs, where oxygen is transferred to the blood. The oxygenated blood is then transported to the left ventricle to be pumped throughout the entire body. Cardiac action consists of repeated cyclic contraction (pumping) and relaxation (filling). Pumping contractions are activated by clusters of specialized cells that generate a bioelectrical signal that prompts the heart's chambers to contract. Both atria contract in unison followed by both ventricles in unison. As the term *bioelectric* suggests, the signals are electric with their biological origins within specialized human cardiac cells that create them. Between signals the heart's chambers pause to relax, which allows them to fill with blood. Theists who argue for a Creator based on the concept of intelligent design most often refer to the complex workings of the human eye as evidence. Why not the complexities of the heart which control life and death? Its built-in electrical system regulates the timing, frequency, and sequence of heart chamber contraction.

A healthy system optimizes the heart's pumping capacity, whereas a deranged electrical system results in generic arrhythmia, which in extreme cases is fatal and one of the leading cause of worldwide cardiac death. Arrhythmia is a generic term that describes several types of abnormal heart rhythm. Ventricular fibrillation, the most prevalent lethal arrhythmia, is a chaotic, continuous, uncoordinated quivering of the heart that renders it incapable of pumping blood. The less frequent form of lethal arrhythmia is asystole. Asystole is an inability of the main chambers (the ventricles) to pump due to the absence of an electrical prompt that initiates their action. The most frequent cause of asystole occurs when the heart's master bioelectrical pacemaker fails to start a sequence of actions that begins with small chamber activation and ends with contraction of the heart's ventricles. Another reason for asystole is failure of electrical transmission from the small to the large chambers, which incapacitates the main chamber pumps. Throughout this book, Stokes-Adams attacks are defined as fainting or near fainting spells caused by transient, sustained, or permanent failure of electrical transmission within the heart's conduction system that results in a heart rate that is inadequate to circulate sufficient blood to the brain.

Arrhythmic death is sudden. Many would-be victims survive because of the swift action of first-response rescuers armed with a closed-chest defibrillator that delivers a high-energy shock to *reset* a quivering heart back to a satisfactory rhythm. Or a first responder may use a closed-chest pacemaker that *jumpstarts* an asystolic non-beating heart by substituting a machine-generated sequence of pulsed electrical energy for the heart's natural bioelectric pacemaker and conduction system. Many patients with markers for arrhythmia, or survivors from sudden arrhythmia death, enjoy extended life with the help of an implanted pacemaker, defibrillator, or a device that combines both forms of electrical therapy. These complex electronic products have two-directional electrodes that *rewire* the heart. The wires route rhythm data from the heart to the implanted device that, after processing, can transmit therapeutic electrical impulses along the same wires back to the heart. Life-threatening situations can be instantly recognized and promptly interrupted by *jumpstarting* or *resetting* the rhythm.

We owe these life-saving technologies to Paul Zoll. Without him, today's 250,000 to 300,000 annual fatalities from sudden cardiac death would be immeasurably higher. Can you imagine what the toll would be without Paul Zoll's discoveries? He caused a tectonic quake with aftershocks when he unmasked the most frequent causes of sudden cardiac death and countered them with emergency electrical therapies to stimulate a heart that would not beat, or to shock a chaotic quivering heart back to normal. The devices that he created were the precursors of today's electrical therapies and of our current emergency cardiac equipment.

Most examples of electric therapies that were applied to the hearts of the apparent dead in the past were poorly documented. A few noteworthy historic examples of these discoveries are presented in the table below. Because Paul Zoll laid a solid foundation for where we stand today, he is regarded by many as the father of *modern* electrocardiac therapy, which is a remedy for life-

Claims of Reanimation By Electric Shock
(See Appendix One for full details)

YEAR	NAME	DISCOVERY	COMMENT
1778	Charles Kite	Cites an archival 1774 account of the reanimation of a three-year-old child by electrical shocks about the body.	Child was likely in a coma, not apparently dead.
1929	Mark Lidwell	Built a portable pacemaker that created a heartbeat with a needle electrode plunged through the chest into the heart.	Reported at a scientific meeting that his pacemaker reanimated a baby.
1929 to 1932	Albert Hyman	Developed three pacemaker models each with a needle electrode plunged through the chest into the heart.	Critics claim that there is no firm documentation of an animal or patient success.

threatening heart rhythms with pacemaker, or defibrillator-mediated electrical shocks. When his widely publicized discoveries were confirmed by other investigators, a worldwide paradigm shift occurred in patient management. In the best tradition of scientific advancement, Zoll's methods were ultimately challenged by newer technologies purporting to have both theoretical advantages and improved clinical outcomes. Yet Paul Zoll will always remain a towering figure among the pioneers who made significant contributions to the understanding and treatment of hazardous arrhythmias. He has a prominent, permanent place in the history of heart-rhythmology for defining and treating arrhythmias with electrocardiac therapy.

Paul Zoll's clinical experience gave him a panoramic understanding of life-threatening arrhythmias. That all-encompassing view led him to systematically approach their early recognition, emergency short-term management and long-term solutions. He lit his candle from the enduring flame nurtured by his predecessors. In turn, Paul's successors lit their candles from his flame and in so doing, they gained enlightenment that has enhanced, and did not diminish Zoll's contributions.

Zoll is most remembered for his medical milestones. He wrote and spoke about their evolution while rarely commenting on non-medical subjects, and he almost never discussed personal issues. Zoll was a very private person – a man of few words. He did not record his personal journey. Nor has anyone else until now.

This book spotlights Paul Zoll as the central pioneer whose contributions extended to the frontier's leading edge of modern arrhythmia management. It also focuses on his predecessors, contemporaries and later day arrivals while telling his private story.

Where did Paul Zoll get the spark of inspiration that led to his discoveries? Let us start at the beginning of his journey.

THREE

BEGINNINGS

On July 15, 1911, a babe was born whose destiny would dramatically change the future practice of worldwide cardiac care. Paul Zoll's parents were hard working Eastern European immigrants of Jewish descent. Hyman Zoll emerged from Pondele, Lithuania. Mollie Homsky's roots were embedded somewhere in Belarus. They met in the United States, married and settled in the Roxbury section of Boston, Massachusetts.[1] The couple was blessed with two sons: Herbert, followed four years later by Paul.[2]

The brothers shared some positive attributes. Both were inquisitive, fun loving, bright and athletic. However, they differed in temperaments and interests. Herbert was an extrovert who pursued literature, music and art. Paul was shy, serious, calm and laconic.[3] His major scholastic interests were mathematics and science. Paul's command of those subjects prompted proud Mollie to volunteer her son's services as a tutor to the struggling children of relatives who needed a boost. Two cousins, David Kaplan and Elliot Mahler, remember that Paul tolerated no excuse for lessons not learned. Their tutor uncharacteristically scolded them, because in his words, "You aren't stupid." Paul later apologized and soldiered on.[4,5]

Paul belonged to an extended family with ten aunts and uncles. Large families were common among Eastern Europeans during the late Nineteenth and early Twentieth Centuries. Hyman Zoll had two brothers and three sisters. All of the Zoll men worked with leather. Hyman and his brother Samuel were in the family leather-goods business, founded in Boston by their father, Shmul. Most clients were in the shoe industry. Hyman's remaining brother, Elias, lived in Cuba where he manufactured woman's shoes. The three sisters were Rose, Chaia, and Lillian. Paul's mother, Mollie, had six siblings. Her twin brother, David, died in Russia. Samuel and Rose came to the U.S.A. Peshe and Hershel immigrated to the portion of Palestine that later became Israel. Mooshy, the remaining sister, is unaccounted for.[6,7]

While Mollie managed the household, she contributed to the family income by being the sole practitioner at her private hair removal service. One room of the home served as her electrolysis treatment center. Mollie was very professional in action and appearance. She wore a short white jacket while ministering to patients who sat on an adjustable reclining chair. Her sons and their playmates were hushed during office hours.[8,9,10] Their silence must have amplified the grisly buzz of each hair root being electrocuted. In later years, Paul attributed his steady hand during surgery to his mastery of electrolysis learned at Mollie's knee.[11] That childhood experience might also explain why bearded men gave him pause.[12]

Mollie and Hyman generously opened their home to relatives who were not fully settled. In return, their live-in guests kept an eye on the boys while Mollie tended to clients or when she and Hyman enjoyed an evening out.[13] The Zoll multifamily home at 71 Walnut Park was typical of the ethnic households in Roxbury and its adjacent Boston neighborhoods of Mattapan and Dorchester. In the early 1900s, Dorchester was home to 250,000 Jews, the greatest concentration in New England. The three communities combined to house the second largest Jewish population in the United States.[14,15] Hyman was observant of Jewish religious practices. Herbert and Paul often accompanied him to services at the Crawford Street Orthodox Shul.[16] Mollie maintained the traditional customs of a Jewish home. The family adhered to kosher dietary laws, honored the Sabbath and celebrated religious holidays. Herbert and Paul attended classes in Hebrew and religious studies. Each had a Bar Mitzvah on or about their 13th birthday to celebrate their transition to manhood in the Jewish community.

Although Herbert and Paul were raised as observant Jews, in later life, both drifted from their formal religious roots. Herbert became a secular Jew.[17] Paul became disaffected when his father, following the traditional orthodox prohibition against autopsy, disregarded his wife's long standing wish for a post mortem examination if the procedure could provide medical information that might help others. Mollie might have had some form of congenital heart disease and had contracted rheumatic heart disease in youth, which was likely a factor in her early death in 1936 at age 49. Paul was a devoted and loving son who wanted to know exactly why his mother had died. But his father considered Paul's arguments for a post mortem examination irrelevant on religious grounds. Thereafter, Paul became detached from institutionalized religion, and conducted himself in accordance with values of humanism that were imbedded in his nature and reinforced during his upbringing in a tight community that placed high value on social support.[18,19]

Herbert and Paul recognized the importance of an education. They were excellent students. Each had hopes of an academic career. Paul followed Herbert to Boston Latin School, a public examination high school located within a block of Harvard Medical School. The entry requirements for Boston Latin were a strong recommendation from a grammar school principal, high achievement on a competitive entry examination and a desire to enter college. Throughout his high school years, Paul – being shy, short and with a suggestion of jug-handled ears – did not participate in many of the community's social opportunities. He did not join a neighborhood youth club, sports team, or the nearby Young Men's Hebrew Association. Yet Paul formed friendships and pursued activities of his own choosing. The teen-ager and his friends celebrated each grade completion with a banana royal concoction at the local ice cream parlor.[20] They welcomed their summer vacation which brought them opportunities to watch the Boston Braves baseball team and gave them more time for tennis at Franklin Field, a large, city-run recreational park and multi-generational meeting place.[21]

Paul graduated from Latin School with distinction in 1928. He followed Herbert to Harvard College, majored in psychology and contemplated a research-teaching career in the field. The tentative plans unraveled when Herbert, an English major, had difficulty obtaining a desirable teaching job in Boston's secondary schools. Mollie, anticipating that Paul would have similar problems, influenced him to apply to medical school.[22] In 1932, Paul graduated Harvard College summa cum laude and matriculated to Harvard

Medical School.

Two important events with future repercussions occurred soon after he began the study of medicine. The first was publication of Paul's undergraduate psychological research.[23,24] The second was his introduction to Dwight Harken, a classmate who became a crucial acquaintance. Their future paths and interests would often intersect. The last year of medical school was one of loss and gain for Zoll. It was the year that his mother died and the year that he gained valuable experience while collaborating on research projects with the legendary professor Soma Weiss.[25,26]

After graduating from medical school in 1936, Dr. Zoll began intense post-graduate training. During internship at Boston's Beth Israel, a Harvard teaching hospital two blocks from the medical school, Zoll managed patients with varied illnesses under the supervision of Herrman Blumgart, Chief of Medicine. He spent the second post-graduate year working and living as a resident in training on the premises of Bellevue Hospital in New York City. While there, the young doctor was smitten by a lovely nurse named Janet Jones. Apparently, Miss Jones did not show the same interest in Paul. The lovelorn physician was so discouraged that he considered transferring to another hospital. As the story goes, when the chief of medicine learned of the situation, he intervened by extolling Paul's virtues to Janet while encouraging her to get to know him better. When she did, Paul resumed work with gusto.[27]

Zoll returned to Beth Israel Hospital the next academic year as a Josiah Macy Research Fellow working with Dr. Monroe Schlesinger, Chief of Pathology. His project was to correlate post mortem coronary artery disease with each patient's pre-morbid clinical cardiac status, to compare the heart after death with the patient's symptoms and physical signs before death. Schlesinger had developed a technique that imaged after-death coronary anatomy with lead agar injected into those arteries, followed by dissection and x-ray of the heart.[28] Schlesinger's insight was a prelude to current day selective coronary angiography first performed at the Cleveland Clinic in 1958 and perfected during the next decade. The technique is performed on a conscious patient and involves advancing a catheter through an arm or leg artery to the entry of a coronary artery that is situated at the base of the aorta, the main artery that carries blood from the heart to the rest of the body. In general the right and left coronary arteries are sequentially injected with an iodinated solution that permits imaging of their inner length and diameter.

The year 1939 turned out to be a period of progress and change for Paul in both professional and personal terms. At Beth Israel Hospital his research taught him much about clinical coronary disease and its complications. Soon after starting to work with Schlesinger, Paul and Janet were married in her apartment in New York City on October 28, 1939. Although Janet was raised in a home of Methodist religious belief, she, like Paul, was detached from her religious roots.[29]

Paul had a penchant to standout, to rise to the top, to be a high achiever. An undergraduate professor's descriptors were "quiet" and "brilliant." Lewis Terman of Stanford University introduced the Stanford Binet IQ test and tracked the achievements of a cohort of high scorers designated by others as "Terman's Termites." The mid-life works of the majority were commendable, but not extraordinary. The few who were most successful also possessed creativity, an added essential ingredient.[30] Paul's IQ scores are unknown. However, a summa cum laude from Harvard College in an era before grade-inflation is equated by some with genius. Yet, as Terman's study showed, that alone is not a ticket to extraordinary achievement. A singular tragic patient outcome merged Paul's intellectual and creative genius on a path to treating life-threatening heart rhythms with electric shock. Dr. Arthur Linenthal, an inner-circle team member, characterized Paul as "a very unusual person…he is brilliant, probably the most brilliant person I have ever known or been privileged to work with." [31]

Other than the one year of training that Paul elected to take in New York City, he was committed to remain in Boston, where most of his time had been spent in the shadow of Harvard Medical School. That pattern would persist for the rest of Paul's life, with the exception of his role in a national crisis of survival. It was now 1941. On December 7th, America went to war. Military duty took Paul far from Boston. He would return to achieve the heretofore unachievable.

FOUR

MEN IN MILITARY SERVICE AND THEIR IMPACT ON MEDICAL ELECTRONICS

Paul was commissioned in the U.S. Army Medical Corps on July 1, 1941. His rank, first lieutenant, demanded physical conditioning and survival training. Past mandatory inclusion on a Boston Latin School precision drill team[1] was a remote memory without value at boot camp. When the military mobilized for war, Janet traveled to be near Paul during his state-side assignments at Fort Oglethorpe, Georgia, and Camp Barkeley, Texas. They parted when he was deployed to Alaska. From there he went to Kiska in the Aleutian chain, which luckily had been evacuated by the Japanese just before American and Canadian forces arrived. Eventually, other enemies appeared in the forms of wind, fog, rain, cold and boredom. When days of limited light and prolonged darkness caused low morale among the troops, the 6th Field Hospital commander reminded Paul that his Harvard University record contained publications in psychology. In the wink of the commander's eye, Paul was made the base psychiatrist charged with boosting morale.[2] Whatever the contributions he might have made, spirits improved with movement of heavenly bodies from the winter solstice that brought a brighter sky and favorable changes in the weather pattern. Paul contracted pneumonia, almost died and was left with a life-long intermittent cough.[3] To avoid a recurrence, the army transferred Zoll from Kiska to the 6th Field Hospital casualty clearing station in England, which was closer to the real enemy.[4]

While Allied commanders finalized plans to invade German-occupied France in 1944, Paul's future was determined by Dwight Harken, a former classmate that Paul had met at Harvard Medical School in the early 1930s. Shortly after graduation, the pair's paths had crossed again briefly when Harken exited New York's Bellevue Hospital just as Zoll entered as a first-year resident. From there the red-head had morphed into a remarkably gifted surgeon. In 1939 he went to England to train under A. Tudor Edwards, one of England's best surgeons. Dwight then returned to Boston, where he remained until the army ordered him to England.

In anticipation of D-Day, the allied invasion of France on June 6, 1944, the military placed Harken in charge of its first specialized thoracic surgical unit at the 160th General Hospital.[5] The facility was on the outskirts of Village Cirencester in the beautiful lowland Cotswold Hills, about 100 miles west-northwest of London. Harken had authority to requisition all necessary equipment for his operating rooms and to hand-pick personnel for his team. He selected Paul Zoll to assist in the care of evacuees with battle-born chest wounds. Dwight arranged for Paul to be transferred to the 160th as his team's cardiologist.[6,7,8] Despite the rigors of his assignment, Paul was so taken by the beauty of the Cotswold countryside that he often described its splendor in detailed letters to his cousin David Kaplan, and no doubt to others. In time Paul became chief of medicine.

Harken's vision of the best way to treat heart wounds was bold, innovative and nearly unprecedented. At the time that Harken was setting up his surgical unit, direct cardiac surgery was banned by Edward Delos Churchill, who had been Dwight's former civilian boss and was his current surgical superior in charge of the the the U.S. medical units in the Mediterranean Theater of operations, which encompassed England at that time. Churchill rescinded his ban on all forms of cardiac surgery after a persuasive appeal by Dwight. With that understanding, the team of Harken, the gifted surgeon, and Zoll, the meticulous manager of intra and postoperative heart rhythms, compiled a remarkable record. During 1944 and '45, Harken removed foreign bodies that included shrapnel, bullets, and debris from within the heart, about the heart and about the great vessels that carry blood to and from the heart. A total of 56 fragments were removed from the hearts of patients, including 12 that were within the right heart chambers and one that was partially within the left ventricle. As shown on the figure on the following page, a total of 136 soldiers were operated upon, incredibly, without a single fatality![9]

Harken's creative approach lends credibility to the adage "necessity is the mother of invention." The surgical team had to innovate because previous reports of similar injuries were weighted towards World War I combatants. In most of those instances, shrapnel that penetrated the heart muscle was managed medically. Rare attempts at surgical removal had met with both success[10] and failure. In a published study in 1939, H. Ryerson Decker mentioned that two patients were operated on to remove a foreign body within a heart chamber; one lived and one died.[11]

After Harken developed the technique of extracting shrapnel and bullets from a heart chamber, he ciné documented his unique operation. The surgeon selected a difficult case to film. Twice before, Harken had failed to remove a nomadic bullet fragment that was migrating between the right heart's large and small chambers. His third attempt would film-document a new, first-of-a-kind, open-heart operation. Success would likely save a soldier's life and might mute the medical establishment's pundits who preached in chorus that a heart chamber should never be entered nor a heart wall violated. On the other hand, failure to retrieve the two-inch metal fragment would label Dwight an adventurous, overly zealous risk taker. With ciné film rolling, Harken entered the heart through an incision circumscribed by an unconventional configuration of sutures designed to prevent excessive blood loss. Dwight would use the same suture configuration in future years in a race for primacy to correct rheumatic hearts with narrowed mitral valves. With Paul Zoll at his side guiding a portable x-ray fluoroscope to image the mobile bullet fragment, Harken succeeded in locating, capturing and removing it in 16 seconds.[12,13]

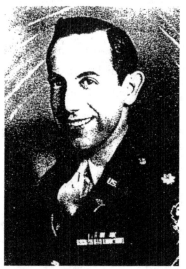

Copy of a photo of Paul Zoll in uniform at an unknown location during World War II. The whereabouts of the original and the existence of similar photos are also unknown. Courtesy of Mary MacIntyre, Paul Zoll's secretary. With permission.

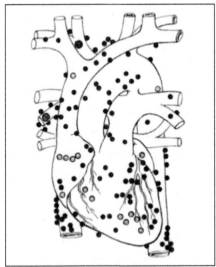

Gross location of foreign bodies removed from cardiac and vascular structures at the 160th General Hospital. Stippled marker show missiles impinging on structures. Black marker shows intrastructural missiles. Crosshatched marker shows embolic missiles. From Surgery in World War II. Thoracic Surgery Volume II. Ahnfeldt AL, Berry FB, McFetridge EM, eds. Office of the Surgeon General, Department of the Army, Washington, D.C. Book prepared and published by Lieutenant General Leonard D. Heaton: U.S. Government Printing Office 1965:354. Also at http://history.amedd.army.mil/booksdocs/wwii/th oracicsurgeryvolIII/chapter8figure144.jpg

The medical establishment must have marveled at Harken and Zoll's breakthrough in a military hospital under challenging, unpredictable and even hazardous wartime conditions. In a letter to cousin David Kaplan, Paul related a lucky experience involving a stray German V-I rocket "buzz bomb" that was flying on target for the Quonset-hutted hospital complex. Fortunately a stiff wind blew the missile off course. The one-ton payload created a deep crater which marred the natural beauty of the countryside that Paul admired so much,[14] but left the hospital unharmed.

While participating in many chest surgeries, Zoll observed that the heart contracted during most manipulations and was extremely sensitive during chamber entry. That lesson would remain indelibly imbedded in his memory and provide a foundation for his ground–breaking work. As Paul later recalled, "I became interested in electrical stimulation of the heart shortly after WWII after I observed much of the pioneering cardiac surgery done by Dwight Harken for removing foreign bodies in and about the heart. The heart responds to stimuli; arousal from ventricular standstill by appropriate stimulation should not be difficult."[15]

In 1946, after serving for five years, Paul Zoll and Dwight Harken left the army and returned home. There they participated in the great post-war realignment of America's energies. Anxiety, fear, uncertainty and worry during wartime were replaced by post-war euphoria energized by optimism and hope for security and peace. Technology was redirected from death and destruction to applications that improved the quality of life. Many inventions, innovations and discoveries from the war had a direct impact on civilian affairs. That included the unprecedented success Harken and Zoll achieved in removing foreign bodies from the heart. Their work continued to resonate some 60 years later. Vice President Richard Cheney accidentally shot his friend Harry Worthington on February 11, 2006. Doctors deliberated on how to best manage a bird-shot pellet lodged in or adjacent to the upper chamber of Worthington's heart. They concluded that the pellet should be left in place even though its irritating presence provoked an episode of atrial fibrillation,[16,17] a relatively benign arrhythmia that did not justify the risk of removal. Likewise, Zoll and Harken carefully evaluated the benefit and risk of removing foreign bodies from the chest of each wounded soldier they treated at the Army 160th General Hospital. Among the total casualties, there was an equal distribution between those who were and were not operated upon.[18]

While some military developments had direct application after the war, many more ideas arose from the large-scale redirection of America's human capital towards civilian aims. An enormous contribution came from The Serviceman's Readjustment Act of 1944, known as the GI Bill of Rights. It offered government-supported retraining in the forms of apprenticeships or undergraduate and graduate education.[19] The massive surge of available manpower at war's end couldn't quickly be absorbed into an industrial workforce transitioning back to domestic production. The benefits of the GI Bill extended for ten-years. "Within the first seven years, approximately 8-million veterans received educational benefits. Of that number, approximately 2,300,000 attended colleges and universities, 3,500,000 received specialized work skill education and 3,400,000 received on-the-job training" according to Daniel Schugerensky in his book *The History of 20th Century American Education*.[20] Tom Brokaw writes in the introduction of his book, *The Greatest Generation*, "The GI Bill was a brilliant and enduring commitment to the nation's future."[21] The GI Bill helped many future luminaries attain highly sophisticated knowledge in the field of electrocardiac therapy. But others, including Paul Zoll and some of his close associates like Dwight Harken, biomedical engineer Alan Belgard and Zoll trainee Milton Paul – who would go on to became a pioneer director of pediatrics – all had career-enhancing experiences while in the military. Other associates, like pacer implant surgeon Howard Frank and electrophysiologist-cardiac pharmacologist Arthur Linenthal, labored on the home front during the war immersed in government sponsored, essential research. Whereas surgeon Leona Norman Zarsky, who later assisted Paul Zoll as his animal laboratory director, filled voids created by the mass departure of her able-bodied male counterparts who entered the military.[22]

Prominent pioneers ascended the ladder of discovery with a direct governmental post-war boost. In the United States biomedical engineers Wilson Greatbatch and Alan Belgard founded major medical electronic firms after they advanced their educations with the help of government funding. In Canada John Hopps became a luminary in advancing his country's electrocardiac therapy program, which likely occurred because he received government assistance in advancing his engineering expertise. Whether participants entered with government assistance or their own resources, the emerging field of electrocardiac therapy attracted the few who were inclined to help the many who suffered from life-threatening cardiac illness. New developments advanced rapidly in a field that was unencumbered by set standards, regulations or federal oversight. Each scientist adhered to his or her ethical interpretation of Hippocrates' dictum, "Do no harm". Paul Zoll started his arrhythmia research without funding. He and other investigators pursued their calling while working in cramped basement laboratories. Some engineers pursued their ideas hunched over a drawing board in a garage or a barn. None complained as they traveled along the road of their dreams.

FIVE

FIRST THE COMMITMENT, THEN JUMPSTARTING A HEART THAT STOPPED TICKING

After the war, Paul returned to an academic appointment at Boston's Beth Israel Hospital which demanded that he serve three masters: the students, the science and the patients. The charge was to teach, to perform original research and to deliver medical care. In the first role as educator, Dr. Zoll taught medical students, medical-school graduates training for specialties, and medical practitioners desiring additional knowledge and skills. Paul became impatient when members of a class, who were expected to be rapid learners, failed to grasp his message. Yet he was very patient and tolerant of groups such as surgical trainees, who had little exposure to most of the information and the issues that he taught.[1]

The obligation to perform original research was fulfilled by resuming pre-war cadaver coronary artery studies. It was a logical choice, because by that time the team of Monroe Schlesinger, Herrman Blumgart and Paul Zoll – now together again – was at the leading edge of understanding the clinical consequences of coronary pathophysiology, and its new, post-war research aimed to further clarify the relationship between specific symptoms and underlying coronary disease. A decade later the standard would become coronary imaging of the living rather than the dead, as it remains today. But by that time Zoll had abandoned cadaver studies to pursue his revolutionary work in life-saving electrocardiac therapy.

In his professional obligation to treat patients, Zoll followed the custom that was common immediately after World War II, when most academics at university teaching hospitals earned their living from private practice. Throughout his career, Paul Zoll maintained a half-time practice that earned him an admirable reputation as a desirable family physician, cardiac consultant and doctor's doctor. His extraordinary insight in diagnosing the cause of symptoms, his management of disease and his advocacy for the ill were accelerants to medical stardom that was an unintended consequence of his deep seated concern for patients. Lael Wertenbaker, biographer of Paul's war time comrade Dwight Harken, wrote, "Zoll was an exceptionally promising cardiologist from Boston, a former classmate of Harken's. He was more interested in patient care than in army rank."[2]

In 1947, a 60-year-old, previously healthy woman suffering from Stokes-Adams fainting spells entered the hospital under Paul's private care. Although the natural history of the illness was unpredictable with a 50 percent annual mortality rate, Zoll was determined to shepherd her to safety. Success depended on intangible good luck and a beneficial response to medication. Neither occurred. Attacks were frequent and prolonged. Zoll and Blumgart solicited advice from other experts. There was no improvement. After three weeks of frantic effort, the patient died.[3] An autopsy revealed a faulty electrical conduction system in an otherwise normal heart. To borrow a phrase used by Claude Beck, the pioneer surgeon who in 1947 was the first to save a life with open-chest defibrillation shock, hers was "a heart too good to die."[4] The tragedy was an emotional watershed that propelled Zoll on his lifelong crusade against arrhythmic death. Diseases that cause tragic death often sow the seeds of their own destruction by rallying forces for cure. Paul Zoll was inspired to build an artificial pacemaker after caring for this vital woman whose sole cause of death was faulty cardiac conduction. Several other exceptional doctors working at about the same time followed a similar course, being motivated by a patient's death or near death from faulty cardiac conduction. Their subsequent discoveries also would sharply reduce the death rate of Stokes-Adams disease.

Within two years, Paul switched from researching coronary disease to exploring electrical management of hazardous arrhythmias. He recalled the experiences shared with Dwight Harken during the war, when Zoll recognized that the exposed heart was contractile sensitive to most stimuli.[5] In addition, the existing literature on the subject contained an occasional fuzzy report of a heart responding to closed-chest stimulation. For example, in Italy, a pulseless dying patient was kept alive for two hours by physician rescuers who rhythmically and forcibly poked their fingers between the ribs overlying the heart.[6] Zoll reasoned that electrical shocks of the proper wave form, intensity and duration might penetrate through the chest wall to arouse an arrested heart.

The project started small, but increased in scale with the support and assistance of prestigious colleagues. They included Dr. Herrman Blumgart, who had shared in the frustration of being unable to save the patient "with a heart too good to die…that only needed a second chance to beat."[7] He encouraged Paul to test the electrical concept and provided research space in the basement of the hospital. Encouragement and needed seed money came from A. Stone Freedberg, a persuasive advocate and officer of the Massachusetts Medical Society, who convinced the research committee to fund Paul's low budget project.

For actual hands-on assistance with the research, Paul recruited Leona Norman Zarsky to direct his fledgling laboratory. She was a graduate of the Massachusetts Institute of Technology, Boston University School of Medicine and surgical specialty training programs in New York and Boston. After her training, Dr. Zarsky had collaborated at Boston City Hospital with Dwight Harken during his pioneering surgical experiments regarding the forced opening of critically narrowed mitral valves that became deformed from rheumatic heart disease.[8] Because Dwight was a task master who demanded total commitment to his workplace, Leona had left that exciting project reluctantly to devote more time to her family. In Paul Zoll, she found an empathetic, recent proud father of twins who understood a mother's commitment to her children. Paul proposed that Leona submit a flexible schedule to accommodate both their research and her family.[9] His willingness to meet her personal needs was rewarded in the contributions she made to the project. Under Leona's tutelage, Alan Belgard, Paul's engineer, learned anatomy and electrophysiology, and Paul's trainees became adroit at surgical technique. Dr. Zarsky developed a simple method to create a permanent electrical heart block in pigs and dogs that was essential for long-term study of pacing electrodes and the Zoll/Belgard "permanent" implantable pacemaker that was to come. The name Leona Norman or Leona Norman Zarsky appears on several of Paul Zoll's most important early publications.

In 1950, the shaky start-up project was in need of an adequate cardiac stimulator that would meet Zoll's expectations.[10] The ideal stimulator – also called a pacemaker – with its electrodes placed on the surface of a patient's chest, would deliver electrical impulses of sufficient strength to reach the heart within. The strength and rate of impulses generated by the stimulator could be precisely controlled by an operator. Zoll never documented any experiments before his "moment of discovery" when he used a borrowed Grass Instrument Company stimulator to pace the heart of an anesthetized dog, although he later implied that he had conducted earlier tests. Therefore the number of experiments, the causes of failure and the variety of stimulators are unknown, except for one comment Zoll made about a small, unworkable, under-powered pacer that was built in-house.[11]

The outlook brightened when Howard Frank, a surgical colleague and friend, invited Paul to attend a session of the American Surgical Association hosted by the Boston Surgical Society, where a Canadian investigator named John Callaghan presented his team's approach to performing open-heart surgery on hypothermic animals.[12] The Canadians had observed that low core body temperatures cause very slow heart rates or an arrested (non beating) heart. Confronted with inadequate time to rewarm a cold heart, Wilford Bigelow, the Canadian team's lead investigator, improvised. He maintained a beat by tapping the surface of a cold heart with a probe,[13] or with generic unspecified pokes,[14] until a native beat returned with rapid rewarming. Bigelow, like Zoll, noted that the heart has contractile sensitivity to manipulation in the course of surgery. Wilford Bigelow also selected electricity as a likely means to prevent or reverse asystolic arrest.

To test that hypothesis, Bigelow called the Canadian National Research Council for help. The council loaned John Hopps, an engineer, to work with Bigelow and John Callaghan, a junior surgeon and the speaker that Zoll heard at the Boston Surgical Society meeting. Hopps' goal was to develop the best method of maintaining a beat during hypothermic heart surgery. The standard method of electrical stimulation on the exposed surface of the heart failed

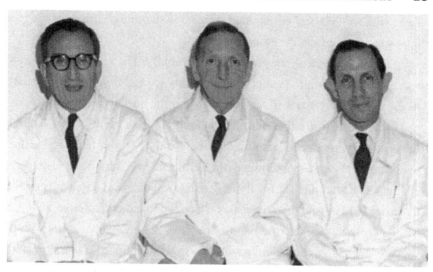

From left to right, A. Stone Freedberg, Herrman Blumgart and Paul Zoll.
Courtesy of Leona Zarsky. With permission.

because it interfered with delicate open-heart surgery by causing extreme cardiac and adjacent muscular movement in the operative field. Hopps solved the problem by developing a bipolar electrode consisting of a thin sleeve that contained two insulated wires within its core. Hopps threaded the tip of his creation through a vein until it reached the general area of the heart's own native pacemaker in the right atrial chamber. The out-of-body ends of the two wires within the bipolar electrode were connected to a Grass stimulator. Hopps' pacer system normalized cold heart action at a controlled rate without extreme movement because the heart was stimulated at low voltage from within. The method became known as *transvenous pacing.*

After John Callaghan finished his Surgical Society presentation, Paul Zoll asked, "What kind of pacemaker did you use?" Although Hopps was in the late stages of developing a new stimulator, Callaghan answered that his group currently used a commercial Grass Company physiological stimulator.[15] Acting on the advice, Zoll borrowed a Grass Thyratron stimulator from Otto Kreyer, who led the Pharmacology Department at Harvard Medical School. Within the year Paul used the device to transthoracically pace the anesthetized dog associated with the initial breakthrough in his basement laboratory. Whereas the Canadian team had directly stimulated the heart from within using Hopps' bipolar electrode, Zoll's 1951 experiment worked by indirectly stimulating the heart with an electrical current that traveled between the surface of the chest opposite the spine and the esophagus.

From that moment, the project moved rapidly. The non-ticking hearts of two patients were started with the stimulator borrowed from Kreyer.[16] Each of its electrodes were attached to a long hypodermic needle carefully positioned just under the skin on either side of the anterior, or front-facing, chest wall. The first patient was paced for 20 minutes before dying from hemopericardium (blood under pressure that surrounds the heart), which was the result of desperate attempts to restart the heart with intracardiac injections of stimulants prior to the arrival of Paul and his pacemaker. The second patient, referred to only as Mr. A, created a seismic rumble by surviving 52 consecutive hours with the support of effective continuous pacing that was discontinued after a slow stable heart rate emerged. When able to function independently, Mr. A was permitted to return home to an uncertain future. He had been under the long-term care of Dr. Freedberg, who related in an interview many years later that his patient had a history of deteriorating health dominated by prolonged unconsciousness, near death and spontaneous revival from intermittent Stokes-Adams attacks. After each spell, Freedberg had questioned if there had been a transcendent episode. The reply was always a *no* – no bright lights, no out-of-body experience and no shadows that resembled ancestors. Just prior to being successfully paced, the patient was admitted to the hospital with yet another near-death experience. A. Stone, already having intimate knowledge of Paul's research, immediately made a referral for consideration of pacer therapy.[17] Dr. Freedberg had endorsed Paul's resuscitation project in the past by allocating laboratory space, finding scarce research funds and inserting pharmacologist-electrophysiologist Dr. Arthur Linenthal as a co-worker into Paul's inner circle.[18] Mr. A's discharge from the hospital to home was an everlasting proud moment for Freedberg. He felt proud to see that his good judgment had resulted in a dear patient's survival, and proud to receive an affirmation of his faith in Paul's vision. The outcome was a powerful endorsement of Paul's theories and method of life-saving subcutaneous transthoracic pacing.

An archival film of Mr. A being paced reveals a comfortable patient with only minimal chest-wall muscular contractions.[19] Unfortunately, that was an atypical and misleading circumstance. After Mr. A, most patients suffered nerve and/or muscle-contraction pain from therapeutic electric shocks. Pain relief was usually accomplished with narcotics, sedation or anesthesia-induced sleep. Although initially misled by Mr. A's pain-free successful recovery, Paul Zoll accepted the risk of producing pacer pain to gain the benefit of preserving life. At the time he had little choice, because it took at least six more years for "reliable" and painless transvenous pacing to emerge as a viable alternative to Zoll's early transthoracic approach. It was also six years before advocates for transvenous pacing found their voice.

Before the transvenous approach became a viable reality, reports surfaced of patients self-terminating transthoracic pacing because they preferred eternal sleep rather than life-sustaining pain,[20] or of a kindly nurse acquiescing to a patient's pleadings to remove the torture machine,[21,22] or of forceful, pacer-induced contractions that threw patients against a wall or out of bed.[23] The situation seemed like a refrain of Mark Twain's comment about the detached doctors who treated his painful gout: "no one knows what hell is like unless they lived there."[24] But unlike Twain's doctors, Zoll "suffered" with his patients. In time, he would reinvent a transthoracic pacer that minimized pain.

After his early success in 1952, there was an immediate need for a dedicated clinical stimulator that would correct the shortcomings of the Grass unit. We don't know much about the borrowed Grass device. Its major deficiencies were marginal power and a design that was inappropriate for Paul's needs. He described it as a Grass Thyratron stimulator and might have omitted the model because it was intended for multifunctional laboratory research. The archival film of Mr. A shows the stimulator with Dr. Zoll's hand adjusting its dials.[25] The instrument does not look like any popular production models of the time. In the year 2006, a long-term employee of the Grass Company was unable to identify the stimulator used in the archival film.

Paul Zoll needed a customized stimulator for clinical use. With headquarters in nearby Quincy, Massachusetts, the Grass Company was a logical choice. Its high-quality stimulators and brainwave recorders were ascending towards an important position in pacemaker therapy. Even though the Canadians did not publish the model number of their stimulator, its image matches one of the S-3 series found in a Grass Company publication.[26] Paul Zoll borrowed a different model that was well suited for sophisticated experimentation in his animal research. He soon learned that it barely met the needs of his early clinical experience. In later years, cardiac surgeon Walton Lillihei would use a Grass stimulator model S-4A in a unique way to drive the hearts of infants suffering the complications of electrical heart block in the aftermath of open-heart surgery.[27] The Grass Company would also go on to manufacture brainwave recording wires that became antennae for the first radiofrequency implantable pacemakers made for thoracic surgeon William Glenn of Yale University in 1959.[28]

Because of the Grass Instrument Company's proven expertise in medical electronics, Paul visited its headquarters with high hopes. He explained his need, revealed his vision and directly asked for help from Albert M. Grass, the founder. Grass might have regarded the presentation as an exuberant flight of fancy about a doomed project. He declined, offering an excuse that the company was operating at full production and did not welcome the prospect of paying more taxes if the Zoll initiative was to succeed.[29] After several more disappointments at enlisting support for a prototype stimulator, Zoll scanned the yellow pages of the Boston telephone directory and called the Electrodyne Company. Alan Belgard, an engineer and co–owner, immediately recognized that Paul's futuristic goals were believable and achievable.[30] Belgard and Zoll became true collaborators. Each started with limited knowledge of the other's field. Alan learned about cardiac electrophysiology and Paul took a course in electronics.[31] Each taught the other. Belgard designed and manufactured an Electrodyne production model transthoracic external pacer that was the first ever intended to succeed in man, as well as all the essential equipment to reverse or stabilize hazardous arrhythmias. The Zoll/Belgard machines became the platform for America's first coronary care unit.[32] Also, the Electrodyne Company manufactured the Zoll/Belgard self-contained long-term pacemaker, which was the world's second device of that class to be implanted. The surgeon was Howard Frank with the assistance of Paul Zoll.

Alan and Paul met frequently. Paul often told Alan of a new need or concept. After further discussions, clarifications and refinements, Alan went to his drawing board. Encouraging trials in the animal laboratory were followed by human trials with Paul as senior investigator. Alan and Paul made adjustments during each phase. If a device was safe and effective, the last phase was production for human use and the benefit of mankind.

In later years, Alan Belgard was asked about the borrowed Grass stimulator that Zoll used in his first laboratory and clinical triumphs. Belgard replied that Paul had success with the stimulator before they met, then added that it was a limited production model intended strictly for research rather than clinical purposes.[33] His view might explain why the machine did not match any publicized production model, was not recognized by a long-term applications engineer employed by the Grass Company and did not match the model S-3 series used by the Canadians, Callaghan and Bigelow.[34] The borrowed stimulator was never returned to Dr. Kreyer at Harvard Medical School because it went missing from Zoll's laboratory.[35]

The ability to jumpstart an arrested heart without opening the chest fulfilled all the requirements for a revolutionary paradigm shift in preventing sudden death.[36] But old-school advocates of open-chest resuscitation, led by pioneering surgeon Claude Beck, resisted change, claiming that their approach was superior while faulting Zoll's approach for being too slow. However, the benefit of closed-chest pacing was confirmed by many investigators and utilized by most practitioners until external transvenous pacing was refined and popularized. The leaders of each school were vigorous in promoting and defending their positions. Paul Zoll found himself in the middle of several fierce debates.

SIX

LASTING FAME AND CONTROVERSY FROM REVIVING THE DEAD

The February 22, 1953, headline of the Boston Evening Post screamed out "Three Dead Brought Back to Life." The article was a confirmation that Zoll's first successful pacemaker reanimation wasn't an anomaly and that additional successes were fulfilling the promise of transthoracic pacing that was first expressed in the editorial that accompanied Zoll's tradition-shattering 1952 New England Journal of Medicine report. The enthusiastic editorialist wrote, "An exceedingly promising report by Zoll in this issue of the Journal describes the successful stimulation of the heart in two patients with complete heart block and cardiac arrest due to ventricular standstill."[1]

Reviving the dead has been a lofty goal of many healers since recorded time. A biblical passage describes Elijah breathing life into a child's limp body.[2] The European Humane Societies of the 18th and 19th centuries were dedicated to rescuing and resuscitating victims of drowning and other calamities.[3] In a celebrated incident in 1777, John Hunter, England's revered scientific surgeon and a member of the Royal Humane Society, plotted to reanimate a popular cleric, Reverend Dodd, after his gallows execution. According to the plan, Dodd's body was to be hastily transported to the undertaker's parlor on Goody Street in London, where Hunter would be waiting to administer electroshock and pulmonary ventilation to arouse the convict. Forewarned prison authorities were determined to avoid embarrassment, so they kept the reverend suspended in death for a prolonged duration. Then, would-be rescuers transporting the body were slowed in transit to Hunter by crowds of the curious and by a heavy rainstorm. John Hunter's efforts were futile. Despite the failure, an apocryphal tale of his success circulated about London. It grew into an enduring myth that Hunter never set straight.[4]

When Paul Zoll began his work on electrocardiac therapy, a vocal minority believed that reviving the dead was against the will of God, or the forces of nature. Albert Hyman, who preceded Zoll as a revitalizer of the apparent dead in the late 1920s, and originator of the term pacemaker, received threatening letters, was named in lawsuits and was confronted by protestors.[5] According to speculation, opposition angst intimidated Hyman so much that he concealed his efforts to resuscitate patients.

Earl Bakken, who followed Zoll chronologically, was also opposed by spiritual moralists.[6] Bakken founded the Medtronic Corporation in 1949. For a brief period, its abbreviated motto was *When Life Depends On Medical Technology*. There is an implication that *Restoring Life* might be included in that broad statement, especially with a corporate symbol of a human figure rising from a supine to a standing posture.

Paul Zoll related that one of his trainees believed that transthoracic electrical resuscitation was against God's will.[7] There were only two trainees at the time, William Gibson and Milton Paul. Fifty years later, when asked about Paul Zoll's recollection, Milton said that he never had a belief system that warranted such a statement.[8]

Still other dissenters did not object on moral grounds, they just doubted that Zoll's methods would work. Within Paul's own medical community, some members did not believe that electrocardiac therapy could be a long-term life sustaining solution to sudden arrhythmic death. In one instance, Janet Zoll, never forgave a doctor at Beth Israel Hospital for his overheard and mistaken negative view of her husband's efforts.[9,10]

Zoll remained undaunted by nay sayers. Leona Norman Zarsky, his research associate, confirmed that Paul expressed confidence in his ideas and tenacity towards achieving his mission. She said that he was seldom troubled by detractors, including unsupportive colleagues or moralists who believed that a preordained master plan was being thwarted.[11] Paul wrote that religious opposition evaporated after a favorable editorial in the Pilot, the newspaper of the Boston archdiocese of the Catholic Church.[12,13] This author attempted to find the specific editorial when conducting research for this book. None that made mention of Paul Zoll or his medical research was found in a search through poor quality microfilm of each edition published between 1952 and 1957. However, a relevant editorial published in 1955 approved of a successful prolonged resuscitation effort on a patient who had a cardiac arrest during surgery.[14]

Criticism from colleagues, medical practitioners and moralists opposed to snatching the near-dead from the reaper was a minor annoyance at best. Zoll's greater concern was deflecting or disproving challenges by contemporary icons. In one case a prominent surgeon named Claude Beck announced that his method of open-chest resuscitation was superior to Paul's closed-chest method. In another case, a research group at the University of Toronto led by surgeon Wilford Bigelow claimed that its pacemaker circuit designed by the team's National Research Council engineer, John Hopps, was copied and not acknowledged in the first, 1954 production model Electrodyne-Belgard-Zoll transthoracic pacemaker.

ZOLL VS. BECK

In the first instance, Paul Zoll's revolutionary closed-chest pacing method to restore arrested heart action challenged the founders and practitioners of open-chest cardiac resuscitation, who had established their approach in 1947 and had solidified their position in the five years prior to Zoll's earliest ground-shaking discovery in 1952. They believed that a rescuer should open the left chest between the fifth and sixth ribs with a blade, thrust a hand inside, and rhythmically compress the heart. In a hospital setting, intravenous or intracardiac medications were often administered in hopes that the chest would not have to be opened to directly pace or administer a defibrillator shock on the exposed heart. Claude Beck was the prime mover and missionary for the open-chest technique. Like Zoll, Beck was a graduate of Harvard Medical School. He had a meteoric rise in the ranks of academia, becoming Chief of Thoracic Surgery at Western Reserve University School of Medicine in Cleveland, Ohio, where he made many innovative original contributions to his specialty.

Claude Beck became a guiding light in establishing the open-chest method of cardiac resuscitation in 1947 when he was the first in the world to restore a life using this approach in conjunction with direct application of cardiac defibrillation. Carl Wiggers, an eminent electrophysiologist and colleague at Western Reserve, had been encouraging Beck to keep a defibrillator in the operating area. Apparently Beck hadn't taken the advice in '47 when he performed his first-in-the-world defibrillation to save a just-operated-upon, 14-year-old from dying by reopening the chest, massaging the heart, and placing an urgent call for a defibrillator. According to reports, the defibrillator arrived either from the far reaches of the surgical suite[15] or from Beck's research laboratory in an adjoining building.[16] Ventricular fibrillation was terminated after several shocks applied directly to the heart.[17,18,19] Future history would reveal similar life-sparing dramas orchestrated by a chest surgeon or cardiologist urgently answering a compassionate call for an experimental or unconventional electrical therapy.

Victims of sudden cardiac arrest have either a total absence of cardiac action or uncoordinated cardiac wiggling and twitching, called fibrillation, which precludes an effective beat. Zoll had a closed-chest pacing therapy for standstill. His 1952 landmark pacing paper predicted that a strong transthoracic electric discharge, administered on the body's surface, could terminate fibrillation and reset the heart's rhythm. Zoll's team started work on an external defibrillator in 1952 but did not perfect the method until 1956. Thus, between 1947 and 1956, open-chest defibrillation was the only therapy. Beck was justified in encouraging physicians to carry a penknife to resuscitate victims of cardiac arrest who had "hearts that are too good to die" or "hearts that have mileage left in them" or "hearts that deserved a second chance to beat."[20] He was evangelical about the technique and collected a cohort of survivors to serve as advocates for it. They were billed as The Chorus of the Dead. Beck organized training classes to create rescuers among the ranks of doctors, dentists and paramedical personnel. Because sudden death occurs at any time in any place, more deaths occur in the streets than in hospitals.

While Beck preached that location was not a deterrent to opening a chest, Paul Zoll focused on responding to in-hospital cardiac arrests. He had a strong conviction that his closed-chest pacing approach was superior to an open-chest approach for several reasons. The closed approach did not require surgical skills. It was without risk of introducing infection and it could be repeated many times on the same patient. Beck had no answer to the question, how often should a chest be reopened? In the event of a mistaken diagnosis of an unconscious patient who had an imperceptible, but present pulse, there was far less harm from transthoracic pacing than from opening the chest. Still, when Paul argued for his non-invasive pacing method at a national meeting, Claude Beck – whose paradigm approach had been in place for nine years – exercised his territorial imperative. According to Zoll, "Beck followed and just wiped up the

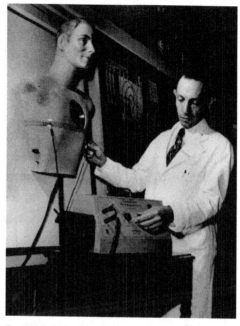

Paul Zoll demonstrates an early model Electrodyne transthoracic pacer on the upper body of a manikin in a photograph taken not long after the first such device was introduced in 1954. Two pacing electrode discs are held in optimal position by an encircling rubber strap. Paul's right hand is near the disc positioned on the manikin's left chest. Courtesy of the Ruth and David Freiman Archives at Beth Israel Deaconess Medical Center. With permission.

floor with me," by insisting that opening the chest was much quicker than placing a transthoracic pacemaker.[21] Yet, Paul made a qualified concession to Beck, agreeing that the chest should be opened after failure of the closed-chest method, but only if assistance is quickly available such as in an operating room, and only if the patient has a good prognosis.[22] It is unknown if Beck ever used Zoll's method. However, in 1960, Zoll commented that he had never opened a chest to massage an arrested heart.[23]

In retrospect, both Beck's and Zoll's approach had faults. The open-chest method lacked simplicity, it often required standby intracardiac medication, and also required an open-chest defibrillator or pacemaker applied directly to the surface of the heart. Transthoracic pacing also required that an appropriate device be available. The closed-chest pacing method lacked assurance that the heart would be stimulated or that stimulation would elicit forceful cardiac contractions. In many instances contractions were too weak to circulate enough blood to the vital organs. Furthermore, in most instances closed-chest pacing created intolerable pain in conscious patients.

In the 1950s, alternatives and remedies to the shortcomings of the two approaches didn't yet exist. A simple method of forcing blood to circulate throughout the body by chest compression awaited discovery, as did development and manufacture of relatively painless, lightweight, portable, and battery-energized pacing devices. Ideal resuscitation algorithms require prompt application by a rescuer. In 1960, a multispecialty group at the Johns Hopkins Hospital in Baltimore, Maryland, discovered a resuscitation method that only required chest compression from a rescuer's hands and oxygen from a rescuer's lungs.[24,25] During the 1960s and 1970s, new technology enabled manufacturers to produce portable, battery-operated pacemakers and defibrillators with reduced bulk and weight.

ZOLL VS. The CANADIANS

The Canadian team of Wilfred Bigelow, John Callaghan and John "Jack" Hopps were remarkably talented. They introduced major advances in the field of heart surgery. It was their 1950 presentation in Boston that inspired Zoll to try a Grass stimulator in his own research. During their exploration of hypothermic surgery, the cold hearts of their experimental animals often slowed and stopped beating. Necessity being the mother of invention, Hopps developed a method to stimulate a barely beating or non-beating cold heart while not interfering with its surgery. He devised a way to pace the inner wall (endocardium) of the right sided atrium (small chamber) with a system that included a semi-flexible bipolar catheter (also called an electrode) and a stimulator, each of his own design. The technique resulted in the first practical method of transvenous cardiac stimulation and was eventually intended to be used in man. The Canadians were also the first to attempt endocardium, inner wall, catheter-based defibrillation of animal hearts, which other researchers would accomplish in humans years later.

Historically, the first electrodes for pacing were enclosed in tubes of rigid glass. In the early part of the 20th Century, Marmorstein introduced hollow glass tubes, termed cannulae, into the jugular veins and carotid arteries in the necks of animals, where they could be carefully routed to stimulate the endocardium of the heart's right atrium and left ventricle. Three platinum electrodes within the glass tubes were configured with one at the tip and each of the remaining two in separate rings near the tip. Any two of three electrodes could be selected for bipolar stimulation from within the heart.[26] By contrast, the flexible bipolar electrode used by Hopps could be threaded through a tortuously meandering vessel.

Bigelow, Callaghan and Hopps conducted their research in laboratory 64 on the basement level of the Banting Institute. Bigelow and Callaghan saw patients at the Toronto General Hospital. These institutions were the major research and medical teaching affiliates of the University of Toronto. Robert Janes, chief surgeon at Toronto General Hospital, recognized that Hopps' system could be adapted to rescue a patient with a dangerously slow or a just-arrested, non-beating heart. Therefore, he encouraged his staff to consider transvenous pacing during their resuscitative efforts on desperate postoperative patients. Apparently, skepticism or inertia among the surgical staff resulted in Callaghan being contacted to jumpstart a heart very late in the resuscitative effort. His attempts to inappropriately, continuously atrial pace five near-lifeless, under-oxygenated, death-bound patients in complete heart block were physiologically doomed from the start because of the patients' sad medical circumstances, and also because Callaghan was unwittingly stimulating the wrong chamber. Callaghan never published the results of his five unsuccessful "honorable failures."[27] In retrospect, long after Zoll's success with transthoracic ventricular pacing in 1952 and Seymour Furman's 1958 success with transvenous ventricular pacing on a patient at Montefiore Hospital in New York, Callaghan reflected that he would have made history had he advanced the catheter two or three more inches from the atrium into the ventricle.[28]

After Paul Zoll's 1952 landmark pacing achievement, the Canadian group complained that he had accorded it only token recognition for its technical help. The impeccable credentials of Bigelow, Callaghan and Hopps lent credence to their accusation. Each expressed unhappiness with Paul in their spoken and printed words.

John Callaghan, in a brief 1980 historical review of the Canadian research group's early experience with hypothermic and normothermic pacing, wrote that after his Boston presentation in 1950, he received a request from Paul Zoll for all relevant data, including Hopps' electrical circuit. The request was honored, he said. "Zoll went on in 1952 to use this for external pacing in a human in complete heart block using external stimulation," Callaghan charged.[29]

Wilfred Bigelow, the most eager team member to pursue his version of justice, confirms in his 1984 book *Cold Hearts* that shortly following Callaghan's 1950 Boston presentation,[30] a letter from Zoll arrived asking for information about Hopps' stimulating apparatus. Hopps and Callaghan eventually supplied Zoll with details, including the National Council of Research circuit diagram. "Zoll forgot to indicate in his articles the source of the electrical circuit diagram that he used in his pacemaker," he wrote.[31] Three years later, the book chapter was reprinted in PACE, the official journal of the North American Society of Pacing and Electrophysiology.[32] In a letter to Seymour Furman, the editor of PACE, following publication of the chapter, Paul Zoll noted that he had properly identified the commercial Grass stimulator suggested by Callaghan during their conversation at the Boston meeting, and Zoll also declared that he had acknowledged Callaghan's help on many occasions. He argued that the stimulator designed by Jack Hopps was not copied and that Alan Belgard independently designed and manufactured the commercial Electrodyne pulse generator.[33]

Four months later, Bigelow answered in PACE that he would no longer debate the matter because he and his coworkers were averse to becoming embroiled in a controversy. Bigelow concluded his letter to the editor on a conciliatory note, "Dr. Zoll's place in medical history is important, unquestioned and secure. He was the first to use a cardiac pacemaker successfully to treat humans and he demonstrated the future role of a pacemaker that was designed and developed for human use."[34] That was a very abbreviated summary of Zoll's achievements. At the time Cold Hearts was published, not only was Zoll credited with being the first to closed-chest pace the heart of man, but also the first to develop alarmed cardiac monitors, and the first to closed-chest defibrillate a human. What's more, Zoll was a member of the surgical team that implanted a fully contained Electrodyne long-term pacer (designed by Zoll and Belgard) into the world's second recipient. He received the prestigious Albert and Mary Lasker Award in 1973 for those notable achievements.

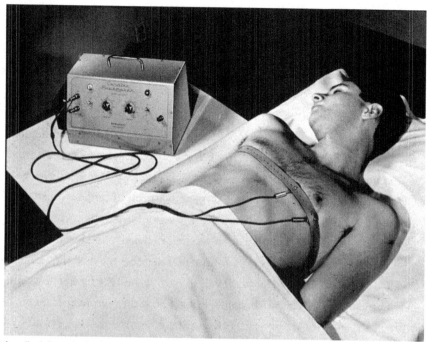

A patient (or volunteer) is attached to an early model Electrodyne transthoracic pacemaker. Both pacing electrodes are on the anterior chest, held in this person's optimal pacing position by an encircling rubber band. Courtesy of Alan Belgard. With permission.

Although the Canadians appeared to back off, by then the dispute had spread far enough to influence others. For example, Äke Senning, the Swedish surgeon who implanted the world's first pacemaker (not self-contained) in 1958, commented in a 1983 summary of cardiac pacing, "In 1952, Zoll introduced an apparatus with a variation of Callaghan's pacemaker circuit. He used it for external pacing..."[35] Even though the apparent public posture of the Canadian group was to discontinue discussing their overt displeasure with Paul Zoll, they did not completely lay the matter to rest. In 1995, John Hopps wrote in his autobiography that "The first U.S.A. stimulator manufacturer did not have a problem patenting his unit which was remarkably similar to ours."[36] [The passage is a likely reference to the Electrodyne Corporation and Alan Belgard, but it is inaccurate because the Electrodyne pacer had no patent.] Hopps pressed on with, "When Dr Paul Zoll of Boston reported his application of our stimulator technique in 1954 [sic], and it opened the door to a new type of heart therapy." [37] [The correct year was 1952.]

Wilford Bigelow, leader of the Canadian team in the 1950s, would grow to become a heart surgeon of immense stature, influence and international impact. He returned to the controversy in a 1996 audio interview conducted by Dr. Seymour Furman, a medical historian and academic surgeon who did pioneering work in transvenous pacing. During the taped interview, Wilfred Bigelow opened a scrapbook containing a letter from Paul Zoll to John Callaghan that requests information about Hopps' pacemaker circuit. Dr. Furman read the letter dated October 30, 1950, reciting, "Dear Dr. Callaghan, I was interested to hear your paper An electrical artificial pacemaker for standstill of the heart which you presented to the American College of Surgeons on October 23. Since I've been working on certain aspects of cardiac resuscitation, I am most eager to get more details of the stimulating apparatus that you used..."[38] Bigelow's clear implication was that Zoll had requested and obtained stimulator and circuit details. In a follow-up interview the next day, Bigelow recalled that upon learning that Zoll was to receive the 1973 Lasker Award at a ceremony presided over by Michael DeBakey, Bigelow wrote DeBakey, "Do you realize that you are giving a prize to someone who had bugger all to do with the development of a pacemaker circuit?"[39]

Bigelow repeatedly expresses his displeasure with Zoll. During a 1991 interview with fellow heart surgeon David Cooper, which was published in 2012, Bigelow referred to Paul Zoll's request, his receipt of information and the Toronto groups' perceived lack of proper acknowledgment. In a vociferous allusion to Dr. Zoll, poorly disguised as Mr. X, Bigelow claimed, "We sent ...an electric stimulator. He then wanted to know how we put it together. We sent him a circuit."[40] Bigelow further claimed that when his team asked the National Research Council (NRC) to patent the Hopps stimulator, they "...went to the patent office where they found it had been patented by the company for which Mr. X had been working."[41] However, Wilford Bigelow's remarks about the patent request at NRC are at odds with that of John Hopps, the inventor of the pacemaker, who wrote, "We were informed that the pacemaker was simply a low frequency signal generator with no novel features in its design or use to justify a patent!" The same office at NRC twice turned a deaf ear to further requests for a patent by the Canadian team.[42]

Bigelow's disparaging attacks must have weighed heavily on Paul. He uncharacteristically bared his resentment during an interview by Alan Weiss on November 17, 1987, the year that Bigelow's chapter accusing Zoll was reprinted in PACE. Zoll explained that "Bigelow, who was a 'big wheel' in thoracic surgery, published a book about hypothermia. Their experiments led them to develop what they believed to be the first pacemaker for which they never got credit because I had stolen it from them." Regarding the claim that Zoll requested information about the Canadian circuitry, Paul said, "I don't remember ever writing such a letter. I looked through my files and could not find it. I spoke to my associates to ask if they ever got any help from Hopps and they told me they did not."[43]

The time line of discovery is helpful in sorting out this controversy. Paul heard Callaghan's presentation in 1950 and was advised that a Grass stimulator might suit his purpose. At the time, the Hopps stimulator was still under development in Toronto. Zoll succeeded in saving a moribund patient with transthoracic pacing in 1951 using a borrowed, unspecified production model Grass stimulator with a thyratron tube. Paul Zoll and his first and only engineer, Alan Belgard, started their collaboration to build their own device for human use after publication of Paul's pacing success in 1952. The first collaborative effort resulted in an Electrodyne production model pacemaker, as shown in the photograph on page 39, that was introduced in 1953, perfected in 1954, and was not patented in the United States or any other country. The unpatented Hopps pacemaker circuit was published by Hopps and Bigelow in 1954.[44]

Alan Belgard unequivocally stated that he never had knowledge of a transfer of technical information from the Canadians to Paul Zoll and he did not receive outside help in building his pacemaker from concept to completion. Years later, after the Electrodyne pacemaker was in production, he was shown a diagram of the Hopps circuit. He said it bore no resemblance to that in the Electrodyne unit.[45] These facts suggest that knowledge of the Canadian circuit did not influence the Zoll-Belgard design. It seems certain that information from the Canadians could not have influenced Paul's first success in human pacing in 1951, because that occurred with an unaltered Grass stimulator. We know that Bigelow showed a letter to Seymour Furman, purportedly authored by Zoll and received by John Callaghan, with a request for information.[46] The

Canadians claimed, but did not present comparative evidence, that their proprietary information or circuit was the same as that used by Zoll, Belgard and Electrodyne.

Although controversy raged, Paul Zoll's success at reviving the dead propelled him to a position of notoriety. He avoided the limelight as he intensified his efforts to prevent sudden death.

SEVEN

FOUND DEAD IN A HOSPITAL BED

The hospitalized ill should not die unobserved and unattended. Yet a patient found dead in bed during early morning nursing rounds was an occasional and even anticipated occurrence prior to the 1950s. Clichés such as "it's a blessing to die in one's sleep," or "a sudden death is the reward for a life well lived," were invoked.

Many of the unattended tragedies were cases of sudden arrhythmic death in victims of acute myocardial infarction.[1] Chances of survival were increased for those under the constant gaze of a limited number of privately paid special-duty nurses. To safeguard patients at high risk to develop a serious arrhythmia, hospitals had an unanswered need for continuous observation of heart rhythm. Fortunately, Alan Belgard and Paul Zoll were well positioned to answer that need. Together, they designed specialized cardiac heart rhythm monitors equipped with alarms for patients who were likely to develop an arrhythmia. Attached to such patients, the heart monitors became sentinels that displayed heart rhythms and gave warning if hazardous conditions occurred.

Along with pacemakers, clinical cardiac monitors were early products of the collaboration between Paul Zoll and his engineer. The devices evolved in complexity over time with added features that provided patients greater assurance of safe passage during a threatening illness. Zoll and Belgard were the first to build clinical monitors for patients in areas beyond the operating room. [2] Alan Belgard's company, Electrodyne, produced and sold the alarmed monitors. The first, in 1953, was coupled to an independent electrocardiograph machine that tracked heart action. The monitor alarmed when adjustable, slow and rapid rate limits were crossed. The Electrodyne monitor's electronics were housed in the same gray metal cabinet that was used for the Zoll-Belgard transthoracic pacemaker. The next iteration was a real-time oscilloscope that displayed beat-to-beat heart rhythm. Another progression instantaneously produced a hard-copy ECG printout of each cardiac rhythm alarm condition. The last generation of monitors reached a pinnacle by displaying multiple patients, each with adjustable alarm limits, automatic printouts of each alarm condition, and each pre/post-alarm rhythm held in memory.

Early in the midst of these refinements in monitoring, a diagnostic-therapeutic advance appeared when Zoll and Belgard coupled a heart monitor to a pacemaker that could automatically activate when heart beats were not detected above an adjustable lower limit.[3] Zoll and Belgard were never credited with primacy for this invention. While all the Belgard-Zoll monitor innovations helped, the monitor/automatic–pacemaker combination, in theory, had the most promising possibility of making unexpected "found dead in bed" incidents a rarity. Indeed, after the Belgard-Zoll monitor initiatives, the incidents of "found dead in a hospital bed" were infrequent. If a patient was on monitor/**automatic pacer** mode, life saving initiation of transthoracic pacing might occur before arrival of a first responder. Thus, Belgard and Zoll developed a second generation of jumpstart machines that could automatically stimulate a heart that stopped ticking.

Aubrey Leatham and Geoffrey Davies were erroneously credited by Seymour Furman, the pacemaker pioneer and historian, as the first inventors of a combination cardiac monitor/ automatic pacemaker.[4] Furman overlooked Alan Belgard and Paul Zoll's solid case for primacy. The issue was never contested by the principals, as was the case with Zoll and the Canadian team of Bigelow, Callaghan and Hopps, who claimed credit for the first human pacemaker of the modern era. Rather, assigning credit for the first monitor/automatic pacemaker combination is a matter for historical correction.

Aubrey Leatham was an outstanding pioneering cardiologist who practiced at the internationally renowned cardiac division at St. George's Hospital in London. He, like Paul Zoll, witnessed the tragic death of a patient in refractory cardiac arrest. Aubrey Leatham was also aware of Paul Zoll's successful pacemaker-related reanimations in 1952[5] and 1954.[6] Because Paul did not identify the model number used in his first success with the Grass stimulator, and because Alan Belgard had not published the circuitry of his unpatented Electrodyne production-model pacemaker that followed, Leatham relied on his ingenuity. He turned to Geoffrey Davies, a St. George's medical electronic technician and charged him to build a transthoracic ventricular-inhibited pacemaker – an approach that had the potential to revolutionize the science of pacing. If the pacemaker could not discharge when there was an adequate heart beat, and would only pace when needed, the device would not fire in the midst of a cardiac contraction's so-called electrical vulnerable period. Pacemaker stimuli that occur during the vulnerable period can potentially cause death as a result of pacer-induced ventricular fibrillation.

Geoffrey Davies had learned electronics while in the service of the Royal Air Force during World War II. He applied his technical knowledge to medical electronics at St. George's Hospital at war's end. Thus Davies shared a similar background with Alan Belgard and other pioneers who had learned electronics while in wartime military service and later contributed that knowledge to electrocardiac therapy. While Belgard had the good fortune to earn his Bachelor of Electrical Engineering degree through the GI Bill at the University of Massachusetts, Davies did not hold a formal degree. Yet he was extraordinarily creative in building both a simple emergency device, and a unique, advanced version in keeping with Dr. Leatham's directive to avoid the electrical vulnerable period of ventricular contraction. This advanced, early monitor/automatic pacemaker combination was credited by Furman to be the first of its kind.

Davies' simple emergency unit plugged into an electrical outlet, but also had an unusual battery-powered back-up system. It could deliver a stimulus with each depression of a hand-controlled telegraph key. The only publication establishing the efficacy of the simple emergency pacemaker appeared in the December 8, 1956, issue of the British medical journal, *Lancet*.[7] The article stated that the simple emergency cardiac stimulator was effective in two patients, gave details of only one of them, and concluded with the revelation that the advanced model could automatically pace a heart that ceased beating for six seconds and would stop pacing shortly, but not immediately, after detecting some native heartbeats. A circuit diagram of the advanced pacemaker that appeared in the report was patent approved by the National Development and Research Corporation three days before publication.[8] However, it is important to note that there is no evidence that the advanced automatic pacer was used in either of the two published cases. The second case was being considered for a more detailed presentation at a later time. The advanced pacemaker went through further phases of development before being manufactured in limited numbers by the firm Firth Cleveland.[9]

The first case in Leatham's British publication involved a 66-year-old woman with a six-year history of Stokes-Adams attacks. Successful pacing was accompanied with extreme pain described as unremitting and unaffected by sedation and narcotics. The report stated that she died during a heart stoppage when the external stimulator was not available. Years later, Leatham revealed that a kindly nurse had removed the pain-inducing pacemaker at the patient's request.[10,11]

A more detailed version of the second case was never published. Furthermore, this author found no recorded cases of success or failure with advanced automatic pacing or its ventricular inhibited function as developed by Davies or Firth Cleveland. However, in private correspondence with this author, Aubrey Leatham indicated that he had non-published successes with the advanced automatic pacemaker prior to his abandoning the entire effort in favor of developing programs for emergency transvenous and long-term pacing.[12]

Seymour Furman's citation of Leatham and Davies' December 1956 publication as factual evidence of primacy is surprising considering his meticulous scrutiny of claims and his devastating criticism of those made by Albert Hyman, who stated that he "saved" animals and humans with his pacemakers fitted with needle electrodes plunged through chest walls targeting their hearts.

Furman knew that Electrodyne developed an automatic pacer. He used the Electrodyne PM-65 in automatic mode on Pinkus Shapiro, the historic first human success with temporary transvenous ventricular pacing.[13] Apparently, Furman did not investigate the provenance of the PM-65 or its Electrodyne predecessors. If he had, he would have been hesitant to claim that the British team was the first to develop an automatic pacemaker. Even Aubrey Leatham was more cautious in stating that he and Davies "might have developed the first demand pacemaker."[14] The issue is important because the evolution of conceptually similar medical electronic devices generally evolve from external large instruments to implanted internalized small devices. Internal machines that **reset, jumpstart** and **rewire** the heart all had an external ancestor.

Alan Belgard and Paul Zoll's proof of concept was demonstrated in 1955 when Belgard linked a cardiac monitor unit to a transthoracic pacer unit. The combination automatically **jumpstarted** the heart of Mrs. Colin McKenzie nine times while she was confined at Boston City Hospital. An image of the patient and the apparatus appeared in newspapers on February 15, 1955, approximately 22 months before the British publication in *Lancet.*[15] Abundant substantive supporting evidence suggests that the Electrodyne automatic pacemaker was in production between the McKenzie trial and the British publication. Correspondence from the Veterans Administration Hospital In Los Angeles, California, to Electrodyne asks when the hospital can expect delivery of the automatic pacemaker and refers to an earlier purchase order.[16] Electrodyne monitor/automatic pacemakers are pictured in local newspaper articles which announce the purchase or gifting of the machines to their respective community hospitals.[17,18] A purchase order from the Mayo Clinic for an Electrodyne PM-65 with electrocardioscope and part No. 113 has been preserved.[19] Electrodyne featured its PM-65 with scope at the October 1956 American Heart Association Scientific Sessions.[20] Paul Zoll and associates first mentioned the monitor/automatic pacemaker in a 1955 publication titled External Electrical Stimulation of the Heart in Cardiac Arrest.[21] It is true that on several occasions when Zoll referred to the monitor/automatic pacemaker's debut, he erroneously attributed its clinical launch to an article published in 1956.[22-26] That being the case, it is understandable that Zoll's misstatement might have confused Furman and others. But in conclusion, there is overwhelming evidence that Electrodyne commercially produced an automatic-pacemaker prior to the Leatham/Cook/Davies December 8, 1956 publication.

Zoll and Belgard might have developed the first automatic pacemaker, but the Davies advanced-design monitor/automatic pacemaker was the first such device to have a ventricular-inhibited mode. Stimulation in automatic-pacing

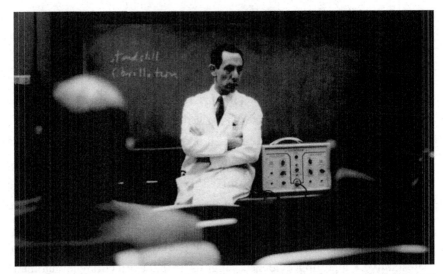

Paul Zoll at the black board teaching colleagues the proper responses to ventricular standstill and fibrillation. An Electrodyne PM-65 cardiac monitor/automatic pacemaker (without oscilloscope) is on the table at his side. Courtesy Ruth and David Freiman Archives at Beth Israel Deaconess Medical Center. With permission.

mode ceased shortly after native rhythm reappeared. In contrast, the Electrodyne automatic unit might operate with prolonged periods of competition between paced and native beats until pacing was manually terminated. In other words, Electrodyne automatic pacing started when there was a need to interrupt a prolonged absence of cardiac action. However, an observer had to be present to manually turn off the pacing when it was safe to do so. Unlike Leatham, Paul Zoll did not believe that competition was a problem or a hazard. In time, Zoll's opinion towards competing paced and native heart beats would re-equilibrate.

It is understandable that even during the introductory era of heart monitoring, families and patients felt reassured by the added security of a surveillance instrument that continuously observed the heart action of high risk hospitalized patients. Some felt so reassured that they went to extraordinary measures to retain the service and felt palpable anxiety if doctors deemed a monitor unnecessary, or ordered that it be removed. In a Boston based case, after a family protested the removal of a monitor from a patient, a relative stole one under cover of darkness from neighboring Peter Bent Brigham Hospital in the mistaken belief that it had continuous therapeutic value.[27] The patient and his relatives were found smiling the next morning after the thief had delivered the monitor to the bedside during the night and insisted that a nurse connect it in working order.

In another unique circumstance, a cardiac monitor had unimaginable therapeutic value when it proved the medical adage that "any mummery will cure, if the patient's faith is strong enough in it."[28] An emaciated hospitalized Haitian man was believed to be terminally ill until an astute doctor elicited a history from which he learned that a Voodoo death curse had been laid upon the patient. Powerful medical energy exorcised the curse after a 24-hour treatment with a cardiac monitor that displayed each heartbeat chirping like a cricket.[29]

A dual-purpose monitor/automatic pacemaker was the centerpiece of a human interest story about Tony Chapelle.[30,31] Conventional or automatic transthoracic closed-chest monitor/pacers were intended for in-hospital use because patients required an array of medical and technical support in the event of a cardiac crisis or equipment failure. Tony Chapelle, who suffered intermittent Stokes-Adams attacks with fainting, was an exception to the rule. He was managed at home supported by an Electrodyne PM-65 with the pacer/monitor leads constantly in place and the alarm condition set at six seconds of asystole. Whenever Tony lapsed unconscious and the alarm sounded, his capable wife turned on the pacing component to jumpstart the heart beat. As he wakened with an adequate heart rate, she terminated the stimulator. Tony's wife must have set the PM-65 on automatic mode whenever she temporarily left the house.

Developments in the engineering of cardiac monitoring were inexorable. An important advance occurred when telemetry technology was developed by competitors of Electrodyne after the company was acquired by Becton Dickenson in 1965. Telemetry permitted multiple patients to be mobile while they wore a small, wireless, battery-operated transmitter that routed data to banks of monitors at a central nursing station. From the start of the Zoll-Belgard monitor initiative, unexpected "found dead in a hospital bed" events diminished in frequency until they became a rarity. Shockingly, in spite of sophisticated telemetry and other advances, properly monitored patients are still found dead in bed because of observer alarm fatigue.[32,33] An April 2013 newspaper article reported that between January 2009 and June 2012, hospitals voluntarily reported

80 alarm-related deaths and 13 serious alarm-related injuries. The voluntary reporting process suggests that the actual number of alarm-fatigue deaths and injuries are higher.[34] Too many alarms and too many false alarms crying "wolf" can result in busy, multi-tasking nurses unconsciously tuning them out in order to deliver essential patient care. If danger signals are ignored, the usual clichés do not bring comfort to bereaved families.

Meanwhile, in another arena, Jack Hopps' 1950 success with transvenous pacing of experimental animals proved to be a theoretical solution to avoiding Zoll's method of painful transthoracic pacing in man. Ten years later, in 1960, Seymour Furman introduced painless transvenous pacing into clinical practice. Following the example of Claude Beck and many other pioneers who resisted change, Paul Zoll vigorously defended his territory. But before moving to that, let us review Paul Zoll and Allan Belgard's progress towards their goal of preventing sudden death.

EIGHT

THE DECADE MIRABILIS: 1951-1960

When Paul Zoll succeeded in electrically pacing the heart of a dog through its unopened chest in 1951, he recognized that there would be a seismic shift in treating hazardous heart rhythms. Zoll later reflected that he foresaw future developments to come during the next 25 years, when electric therapy would outperform, supersede, and complement standard drug management.[1] His prophetic insights depended on coming technical advances that would germinate dormant theoretical solutions such as closed-chest defibrillators and implantable long-term pacemaker systems. It took a decade for Zoll's creative solutions to be birthed and for Alan Belgard to transform Zoll's stated needs into practice and public awareness. Belgard seized upon adaptable new science and technology as they emerged, incorporating the new discoveries into electrocardiac diagnostic or therapeutic instruments. It was a *decade mirabilis*, a decade of miracles.

The term *annus mirabilis*, year of miracles, is more common. Albert Einstein had his *annus mirabilis* while working as a patent inspector in Bern, Switzerland. In 1905, during his spare time, he wrote four manuscripts. Each was a theory of principle postulating rules that all natural phenomena must satisfy. They revolutionized concepts of time, space, matter and energy.[2] The first described the nature of light and laid the foundation for quantum physics. The second related to molecular and atomic collisions in a way that explained Brownian motion, or the apparent movement of particles. The third involved the speed of travel relative to the speed of light. It was known as *The Special*

Theory of Relativity. The fourth explained that energy and matter are related and was expressed in the famous formula, $E=MC^2$.

If Paul Zoll merely had to theorize his four major discoveries, the decade-long incubation of his ideas would have been markedly compressed. The 1952 transthoracic pacer success in man might have occurred in 1950 or 1951, and the alarmed cardiac monitor, transthoracic closed-chest defibrillator and fully implantable pacemaker would have followed in rapid succession. But Zoll had to wait for technology to catch up with his vision. During the decade, vacuum tubes were displaced by transistors, small mercury-zinc battery cells supplanted larger batteries, and bulky instruments were miniaturized. The road to success was tortuous.

The application of incremental advances in technology between 1950 and 1960 required the patience of Alan Belgard, who was Paul's only engineer and 16 years his junior. He, like Paul, was born and raised in the Roxbury-Dorchester district of Boston. Their homes were 1.4 miles apart. When Paul was serving as a doctor in the U.S. Army toward the mid-point of World War II, Alan was in high school. At the time, the government sought to fill its need for personnel skilled in electronics by sponsoring a program for high school students to spend half-time at a certified electronics school. Young Alan enrolled, and later graduated high school with a major in radio and electronics. He then enlisted in the Navy in 1945. Alan's recently acquired background in basic electronics qualified him to attend an advanced military electronics school for a year of training in radar and sonar. After his discharge from active duty in 1946, he turned to the GI Bill as his pathway to a college degree in electrical engineering. Alan considered applying to the Massachusetts Institute of Technology (MIT). When he learned that MIT had already selected its entering classes for the next three years, Belgard applied to the University of Massachusetts and graduated with its first engineering class in 1950. Between 1950 and 1952, Alan worked as an engineer for the American Machine and Foundry Company designing and maintaining training equipment that simulated the gunnery on a B-29 Super Fortress.[3] Then, he and two partners bought the bankrupt Electrodyne Company for its debt. They resuscitated the company with a variety of electromechanical devices that measured nerve stimulation-muscle response time.

When Belgard and his partners were reviving Electrodyne, Paul Zoll was gaining greater awareness of the inherent inadequacies of the Grass stimulator he used to closed-chest pace the hearts of his first published patients. He needed a customized pacemaker, so Zoll contacted the Grass and Sanborn companies, among others. When none believed that his plan would have a successful outcome, Paul went to the telephone directory, in a seemingly quixotic quest, where he found Electrodyne listed under the heading *Physiological Stimulators.*[4] Paul called, spoke to Alan and they arranged a meeting, at which Belgard immediately seemed to grasp the potential of Paul's vision and needs. The two became long-term collaborators. Rather than redesign the Grass stimulator that Paul had borrowed from Otto Kreyer, Alan started from first principles. He had a working prototype within months and made serial improvements during the next 18 months before Electrodyne marketed its first 27A production model. Many successful products followed from their teamwork during the periods when Alan Belgard was chief engineer of Electrodyne, from 1952 to 1956, and president from 1956 to 1965.

Paul and Alan forged an extraordinary and enduring collaborative bond that delivered four valuable gifts to mankind during their most productive decade: the transthoracic pacer, alarmed cardiac monitor, transthoracic closed-chest defibrillator, and fully implanted pacemaker. They worked as true partners, constantly exchanging ideas, sometimes disagreeing, but always driving towards a common goal. When one of Paul's theoretical needs was transformed into practice, Alan Belgard received Paul's praise and credit.

Meanwhile, the decade percolated with post World War II scientific achievements and political tensions. The U.S. and Russia were locked in a cold war. America detonated the first hydrogen bomb in 1952. Russia caught up shortly thereafter. Commercial jet airline service began in 1957. The Russian aerospace program launched Sputnik, the first Earth-orbiting satellite, the same year.

At the same time, back on earth, Seymour Furman, then a trainee at Brooklyn's Montefiore Hospital, succeeded in pacing the right ventricle of a dog in a subterranean basement laboratory. In 1958, Furman and the Montefiore team scaled a previously unreachable summit when they stabilized a Stokes-Adams patient by using transvenous ventricular pacing.[5] Pincus Shapiro smoked a celebratory cigar as he was discharged from hospital to home after having the pacer electrode in place for 96 days.[6] Furman's achievement presented a powerful challenge to Paul Zoll and his method of transthoracic emergency cardiac rescue, established more than half a decade earlier.

NINE

EMERGENCY TRANSVENOUS VENTRICULAR PACING, AN ALTERNATIVE TO TRANSTHORACIC PACING

An elderly man entered New York's Montefiore Hospital on June 27, 1958, with a history of frequent syncope. A marginal heart rate had resulted in fainting spells and multi-organ failure. The patient, Pincus Shapiro, was treated with rate accelerating medications and a transthoracic Electrodyne pacemaker bearing the words "Developed by Paul M. Zoll, M.D." But Shapiro's need for intermittent pacing provoked intolerable pain, which persisted after doctors administered narcotics and sedatives. To minimize discomfort, a private-duty nurse jumpstarted the heart when it stalled and inactivated the pacer when spontaneous heart activity returned.[1] If Shapiro's pathetic condition did not improve, the physician team, led by John Schwedel, had a radical new rate stabilizing option. It was a work in progress at Montefiore Hospital under the direction of senior trainee Seymour Furman. His concept, known as transvenous pacing, was to insert an electrode catheter into a vein and advance it to the right-side main heart chamber (right ventricle). The out-of-body end of the electrode was connected to a model P27A Electrodyne pacer fitted with a voltage-reducing adapter that Furman designed to modify the system for internal cardiac stimulation. Transvenous pacing eliminated both the need to open the chest and the potential pain that accompanied pacing the heart from the surface of the chest. The approach was somewhat similar to the one developed by Jack Hopps in Toronto using an advanced design bipolar catheter in animals. But Furman was unaware of Hopps' work. At Montefiore, the system had already worked in animals and during one surgical procedure in a high-risk patient.[2,3]

Sudden deterioration in Shapiro's condition triggered the contingency rescue strategy. When Seymour Furman's wife received an urgent call at her home, she located a custom built unipolar electrode in a bureau drawer and hurriedly became the courier to Montefiore. An immediate attempt to insert the catheter at the bedside failed. However, success was achieved in the hospital's x-ray suite the next day, August 18,1958.[4] Painless transvenous pacing eliminated the need for narcotics and sedation. At first, a private duty nurse turned the model P27A stimulator on and off as needed, until the Shapiro family donated an advanced model Electrodyne pacer that could operate automatically. The PM-65 also bore the inscription "Developed by Paul M. Zoll, M.D." It incorporated a cardioscope that continuously displayed heart rhythm. Another feature was a menu of pacing-mode selections that included *External, Internal* and *Automatic*. The last, *Automatic*, was the mode chosen to transvenously jumpstart Shapiro's heart after each five-second asystole. The PM-65 was large and heavy. It moved on wheels and was line powered from a wall outlet.

Furman was also unaware that, in Minnesota, Earl Bakken had invented a small, transistorized, and battery-operated cardiac pacemaker at the request of Walton Lillehei at University Hospital in Minneapolis, Minnesota. Many of Lillehei's pediatric patients, following corrective surgery for congenital heart disease, suffered the complication of "heart block" in the immediate postoperative period. Their slow heart rates required pacing. Lillehei had asked Bakken to create a battery powered unit following the death of a child who had been dependent on a line powered pacer that failed during a prolonged area-wide electrical power outage.[5] Bakken's design was inspired by an article in Popular Electronics magazine.[6] To accelerate and stabilize the slow heart rates of Lillehei's patients with heart block, a Bakken pacemaker was attached to the out-of-body end of a thin wire electrode. Lillehei loosely attached the other end of the electrode to the surface of each surgically resurrected heart during the finale of his operation. It was later removed, but in the critical post-operative period, the electrode stood ready to deliver pacing to children who would need it.

At Montefiore Hospital during that late summer and early fall of 1958, Pincus Shapiro languished in constant need of his transvenous pacer for life support. The family requested a second opinion from an acknowledged expert in the field. By coincidence, Paul Zoll, an upper tier choice, was at a medical meeting in New York City. Schwedel, Shapiro's lead physician, escorted Zoll to Montefiore for a consultation. After a lengthy review of the record and examination of the patient, Zoll disparaged the approach taken by the Montefiore team. He declared that the transvenous pacer was a danger and enumerated a number of problems that might occur, such as catheter electrode displacement with failure to pace, the introduction of infection through the catheter electrode entry site, and catheter perforation of the heart wall – each was a good reason to remove the pacing electrode in advance of a complication.[7] Zoll then left without suggesting a clear alternative. Schwedel and his team disregarded Zoll's objections and Pincus Shapiro stayed the course with his heart rewired with a temporary transvenous electrode, stabilized in frail but better health, and returned home for Thanksgiving after 148 days in Montefiore with transvenous pacing assistance somewhat less than the 96 days in which the catheter electrode was in place. With a celebratory cigar between his lips, Pincus departed in a shower of publicity and fanfare.[8] Mr. Shapiro represented as great a personal accomplishment for Seymour Furman as Mr. A. had been for Paul Zoll at Boston's Beth Israel Hospital six years earlier following 52 consecutive hours of external transthoracic pacing.[9]

The Furman/Zoll interaction had a thorny postscript. Furman and Schwedel's manuscript describing their transvenous pacing success was rejected by the New England Journal of Medicine. Through subtle clues, Furman believed that Paul Zoll was the referee who judged the manuscript unworthy of publication. That gave Furman grounds to appeal the unfavorable decision. Paul Zoll should have recused himself because of prior direct involvement with the patient.[10,11] After a favorable appellate review, the paper was published.[12] The article's initial rejection must have marked a second instance when Seymour Furman was offended by Paul Zoll's unfavorable opinion of emergency transvenous pacing. After Zoll's appearance at Montefiore, trainees were cautioned to only whisper his name.[13]

Zoll never mentioned that "his" P27A and PM-65 stimulators powered the first successful transvenous pacing system in man, even though the procedures were initiated without his knowledge and the PM-65 was continued against his wishes.

Whenever Zoll revisited the issue of emergency transvenous pacing, his views were unchanged, sincere, fixed and without apparent animus toward Furman. In time, Zoll would improve upon his method of emergency jumpstarting the heart by external transthoracic pacing.

During the time between his own and Furman's historic accomplishments, Zoll had long since succeeded in jumpstarting would-be fatal heart rhythms with closed-chest pacing. Zoll had also been the first to succeed in resetting would-be fatal heart rhythms with closed-chest defibrillation in a closely contested, and somewhat controversial, race to lead the world.

TEN

CLOSED-CHEST DEFIBRILLATION: ANOTHER WAY TO REVIVE THE NEAR DEAD BY RESETTING HEART RHYTHM

In 1952 Paul Zoll predicted that high-energy transthoracic electric shock could save a person in ventricular fibrillation by resetting the rhythm of the heart.[1] He made that prediction a reality in November 1955 by preventing the death of a patient with an Electrodyne line-operated alternating-current defibrillator. The patient, known as "case number four," seemed blessed like Lazarus. He "rose from the dead," and walked out of Boston's Beth Israel Hospital to celebrate Christmas with his family. Zoll's remarkable achievement was presented to the medical world in an April 1956 issue of The New England Journal of Medicine.[2]

Although Zoll was the first to shock a human back to life without opening the chest, his breakthrough had precedents. Even pre-20th Century history records numerous pronouncements about the medical possibilities of electrocardiac therapy. One claim in particular merits serious consideration. In 1775 Peter Christian Abeldgaard, a Danish physician-veterinarian working in Belgium, performed a set of experiments that encouraged further investigations into the cause of electrical death and revival. Abeldgaard released electrical energy, stored within Leyden jars, to the heads of six hens. All promptly fell motionless to the ground. Abeldgaard then shocked the chests of three, returning them to normal activity in sharp contrast to the three motionless hens that were denied a second shock.[3] Were the apparently lifeless fowl in a state of suspended animation, deep coma or were they dead? To answer the question, Abeldgaard repeated the first phase of the experiment on two hens, but this time he left the newly inanimate birds undisturbed, with no second shock to the chest. He returned the next day to find them stone cold and stiff from rigor mortis.[4] The intuitive, but unproven, construct was that the first shock to the head caused ventricular fibrillation as the electrical current traveled to ground. The second shock to the chest of the three hens that survived reset their fibrillating hearts back to normal. In Denmark, Abeldgaard's observation is considered the first demonstration of cardiac defibrillation.[5]

More than 100 years later, in 1887, John MacWilliam, a British researcher who was born, studied and worked in Scotland, proved that a low-intensity cardiac electroshock provokes ventricular fibrillation in open-chest animals.[6] Shortly after that, he drew upon evidence and experience to propose that the leading cause of sudden death in man was ventricular fibrillation. MacWilliam further proposed that such fibrillation might be reversed by a high-energy electric shock delivered through properly positioned paddles across a closed chest.[7] That was in 1889, but no one acted to prove or disprove the theory. Yet in the same year, two French investigators, Jean-Louis Prevost and Fredric Battelli, working in Geneva, demonstrated that a weak electrical shock applied directly to an animal's heart caused ventricular fibrillation that was reversed with a second shock of higher intensity.[8]

In the 20th Century, Carl Wiggers, the iconic physiologist at Western Reserve University in Cleveland, Ohio, proved through verifiable scientific experimentation that a properly timed electroshock to the exposed heart provokes ventricular fibrillation and that a second "countershock" resets the heart back to normal rhythm, providing a scientific foundation for the Abeldgaard construct of 1775. It was Wiggers who prepared Claude Beck for the epochal first human success of open-chest ventricular defibrillation in Cleveland in 1947. Before that, Wiggers had been a dissenter. He had doubted the credibility of Prevost and Battelli until three Americans, Donald Hooker, William Kouwenhoven and Orthello Langworthy, published an account of their open- and closed-chest animal experiments that confirmed Prevost and

Battelli's findings.[9] Wiggers reconsidered his objections, reversed his thinking and followed suit with his own research in electrocardiac therapy while receiving financial support from the Rockefeller Institute and Consolidated Edison.

For all his accomplishments, Wiggers also exemplified how knowledge is of limited value if it is inaccessible or disbelieved. Exposing a mind-set similar to his dismissal of the Prevost and Battelli findings, Carl Wiggers acknowledged that he had prejudged that the heart could not be paced or defibrillated through a closed chest.[10a,10c] There is little doubt that Wiggers, charged with determining the merits of scientific projects in search of U.S. government grant support, blocked approval of Paul Zoll's grant application. Zoll himself described the culprit as "An eminent physiologist from Cleveland...who decided that our success was not possible because he had failed with similar experiments 20 years earlier."[11]

Despite such resistance, the stage was set in the western world for a therapeutic advance of massive proportion. William Kouwenhoven, Paul Zoll and Arthur Guyton had already succeeded in closed-chest ventricular defibrillation of animals. When Zoll was well into his own animal research, he likely learned of many similar successes in Russia involving Nuam Gurvich's use of alternating and direct-current devices.[12,13] Leona Norman Zarsky recalled an excited Paul Zoll bursting into the laboratory after he had learned that large animals had been successfully closed-chest defibrillated in Russia.[14] Who would be the first to closed-chest defibrillate a human?

Zoll was fully prepared and anxiously awaiting a patient to defibrillate and to eventually send home from the hospital intact – the gold standard for a successful outcome. That hope was realized in the personage of case number four, as the patient is listed in Zoll's first published series on human defib-rillation,[15] shown on page 63. The 67-year-old man entered Beth Israel Hospital on November 17, 1955, with intermittent fainting spells from brief episodes of non-sustained rapid ventricular heart action. He had a history of recent syncope from both excessively rapid and slow heart rates. If his racing heartbeat did not stop, if it degenerated into ventricular fibrillation, or if there was dual instability from too fast or too slow a heart rate, case number four might die. During the first night in a high-level surveillance unit, a dreaded episode of ventricular fibrillation was successfully shock terminated *(reset)* by Victor Gurewich, the in-house medical resident. Victor dutifully followed the common custom of documenting arrhythmias and interventions by recording the hour, minute and sequence of each event on the patient's real-time electrocardiogram (ECG). During morning report, while Zoll listened impatiently, Gurewich described the snatch from the jaws of death back to life. Zoll waited with hand outstretched to receive the proof in the form of facts written on the two-and-a-half-inch-wide, ribbon-like ECG paper that would substantiate Gurewich's narrative. When Victor finally placed the evidence in Zoll's palm, the young trainee expectantly awaited praise for a job well done, but Zoll frowned as he scrutinized the dramatic evidence. His tight lips parted and he said, "I am going to have trouble publishing this data. Why did you write all over the ECGs?" He then abruptly turned to see the patient.[16] Although most of the entries were trimmed from the margins of the paper, a few handwritten characters remained on the edited ECG tracings that were published.[17] (See panel B in photo on facing page.)

During recovery, the patient made two demands. He wanted to have traditional Italian food and he wanted to be home in time to celebrate Christmas. His dietary request was met by his obliging family, yet the fulfillment of the Christmas wish was uncertain because of cardiac instability marked by progress and setbacks. Improvement plateaued at marginal levels. Ultimately, all that could be done had been done, so it was "home for Christmas" with Dr. Zoll's blessings. There are conflicting versions of what followed. The original New England Journal of Medicine case report states that the patient was still living three months after discharge. Zoll later mentioned that death occurred three months after leaving the hospital.[18a,18b] In fact, the patient died suddenly at home two and a half years after being released to celebrate Christmas. During the long interval, he suffered repeated fainting spells that required frequent hospitalizations. After two years, "number four" had endured the application of approximately 100 countershocks for ventricular fibrillation.[19] This courageous man exemplified the natural course of many of the ill who are given the choice of trying an untested, potentially life-saving treatment, or choosing to prepare for certain death in the short term. As defibrillators developed in the 1950s, many such patients were winning the battle while hospitalized, but losing the war after discharge – hopefully in the comfort of their own homes. Clearly the long-term stabilization of life-threatening, hazardous heart rhythms was needed. Solutions by Dr. Paul Zoll and other medical pioneers were already in the works.

In the meantime, the other investigators pursuing closed-chest defibrillator therapy met with mixed

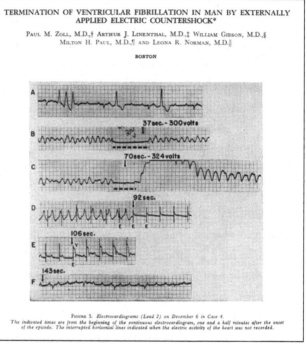

TERMINATION OF VENTRICULAR FIBRILLATION IN MAN BY EXTERNALLY APPLIED ELECTRIC COUNTERSHOCK*

PAUL M. ZOLL, M.D.,† ARTHUR J. LINENTHAL, M.D.,‡ WILLIAM GIBSON, M.D.,§ MILTON H. PAUL, M.D.,¶ AND LEONA R. NORMAN, M.D.‖

BOSTON

FIGURE 5. *Electrocardiograms (Lead 2) on December 6 in Case 4. The indicated times are from the beginning of the continuous electrocardiogram, one and a half minutes after the onset of the episode. The interrupted horizontal lines indicated when the electric activity of the heart was not recorded.*

Title page from the New England Journal of Medicine with insert of heart rhythm strips of patient # 4 that demonstrate successful countershock, or high voltage closed-chest defibrillation and pacing. Complete citation, Chapter 10, reference #4,Copyright 1956. Reprinted with permission from the Massachusetts Medical Society.

results. Arthur Guyton published only one report of success in experimental animals and postulated that closed-chest defibrillation of humans was possible.[20] William Kouwenhoven went much further.

One and a half years after Zoll's first success and eleven months after his transforming publication, Kouwenhoven succeeded in defibrillating a patient using a line-powered, alternating-current unit that he invented at Johns Hopkins University in Baltimore, Maryland.[21a,21b] Kouwenhoven was an eminent senior pioneer with long experience and accumulated wisdom that dated to 1926, when he committed to find a way to save electrocuted linemen who worked for Consolidated Edison. At the time, America was rapidly becoming electrified, with street lamps replacing gaslights and homes glowing from brightly illuminated incandescent bulbs. The transition was apparent as early as 1893 when the Chicago World's Fair was ablaze with light symbolic of the revolution in progress. Kouwenhoven was an electrical engineer by training and in practice. In addition, he proudly held an honorary degree in medicine bestowed by Johns Hopkins University for his significant contributions to medical electronics. He also exhibited some distinctive personal preferences, such as keeping a tobacco pipe as a constant companion and living on his sailboat on the Chesapeake Bay during summers.[22] In 1953, when Consolidated Edison asked Kouwenhoven to develop a closed-chest defibrillator, he knew that an electrocuted lineman dying in ventricular fibrillation could not live long enough to be transported to hospital without some form of yet undiscovered or unremembered life support. He knew that a portable direct-current defibrillator had to be available on-site to save a dying victim. The inventor-sailor incorporated that conceptual knowledge into a defibrillator powered by either line current or a truck battery.[23] Co-workers at Hopkins later stated that he might have succeeded in defibrillating a human before Paul Zoll if Alfred Blalock, Chief of Surgery at the hospital, hadn't insisted on extensive and convincing evidence of animal survival prior to attempting transthoracic defibrillation on a patient.[24,25]

Even though Blalock might have delayed a Kouwenhoven-inspired human trial and publication, a great good was achieved from the meticulous animal experimentation he insisted upon. Life-sparing manual chest compression was rediscovered by Kouwenhoven and his associates, resurrecting a method of external cardiac massage similar to those first recorded in Germany in the late 1800s and practiced into the early 20th Century, at which time such methods were inexplicably abandoned.[26-28] The methods were the distant forerunners of today's cardiopulmonary resuscitation (CPR).[29]

A challenge to Zoll's primacy arose as recently as 2009, when a report surfaced that a Russian team led by Nuam Gurvich succeeded in closed-chest direct-current defibrillation of humans in 1952, three years before Zoll's first success with case number four.[30] It is a fact that brief English-language summaries of Gurvich's early work with closed-chest defibrillation of animals had appeared in 1946 and 1947. At that time, he had predicted that the procedure would work in man.[31,32] But no firm citation records when his prophecy materialized, what occurred or where in the Soviet Union the exhilarating event took place. Evidence indicates that Russian defibrillators capable of the task existed in 1952. The 2009 report makes reference to 1959 Soviet Ministry of

Health guidelines that further reference a 1952 guideline requiring that all operative areas in major hospitals have a direct-current defibrillator.[33] A Russian made, Gurvich inspired, relatively compact production model direct-current defibrillator, circa 1952 was brought from Russia to Cleveland by Dr Robert Hosler in 1958. The device is currently displayed at the Dittrick Medical History Center, Case Western Reserve University.[34] Although Hosler brought back a defibrillator, he did not bring back knowledge that patients had been defibrillated between 1952 and 1958. American scientist Guy Knickerbocker worked for three months in the Soviet resuscitation laboratory of Vladimir Negovsky, where Nuam Gurvich was the leading researcher. Neither Gurvich, nor anyone else, informed Knickerbocker of the 1952 achievement.[35] It is similarly remarkable that Negovsky, in a 50-year review of achievements at the Institute of General Reanimatology, does not specifically mention that Gurvich succeeded in closed-chest human defibrillation, only that "Gurvitch [sic] helped to design the first commercial defibrillators which appeared in the USSR in the early 1950s."[36] At a later time, Bernard Lown – who can claim to be the first to introduce emergency, closed-chest, direct-current defibrillation and was the first to introduce elective cardioversion (non-emergency shock to correct arrhythmia) into clinical practice during the 1960s – visited the Soviet Union on several occasions, and partnered with Eugene Chazov, Director of Moscow's Soviet Cardiac Research Institute, on projects of mutual interest.[37] Apparently, Lown was not informed during his first Moscow meeting in 1972 that he had been pre-empted by Gurvich's successful human reanimations with direct-current defibrillation.

The Russian claim of early transthoracic defibrillation raises many questions. Did anyone in the western world possess or have access to that knowledge? Assuming that the claim is true, why did Russia fail to share this important information with the West? Did Soviet authorities consider their defibrillator and its application a state secret during the Cold War? Did doctors lack incentive to publish because advancement in the Soviet medical system was not necessarily based on merit?

Whatever the answers, the Russian achievement was not publicized, is not well documented, lacks the time-honored necessary data to withstand scientific scrutiny, and apparently did not result in an extensive transformation of customary practice. That accolade remains with Paul Zoll. Claims about Gurvich's achievements in Russia by Ivan Cakulev and colleagues after more than a half century latent period[38] are extremely important, but they do not diminish the contributions of Zoll. Until the lingering Russian fog of the Cold War can be penetrated to reveal the circumstances of that country's human reanimation experience with closed-chest defibrillation, Paul Zoll holds the verifiable scientific credentials to retain his position as the first to save a patient using transthoracic defibrillation.

Paul was the prophet and master of transthoracic defibrillation technology as it gained momentum to become firmly established through the late 1950s and early 60s. Defibrillators that salvaged patients on the brink of death became commonplace. Throughout that period, survivors were no longer a rare medical curiosity. In the early 1960s, long-term implantable pacemakers were still in their infancy. They too were destined to grow in popularity and become widely accepted.

Even though defibrillator use became commonplace, each "save" by those devices remains laced with human interest and each adds an inspirational story to our human experience. Some of the stories are more memorable than others. "God was looking over his shoulder" is an oft repeated aphorism that is grounded in faith. The aphorism also reflects the fact that patients are always willing to accept offers of extra "help" because they recognize that medical outcomes are uncertain, even with advanced technology and highly trained personnel. While on a hospital pastoral visit, a priest was stunned when his parishioner-patient slumped over unconscious from a Stokes-Adams attack. The priest immediately called for assistance. After successful defibrillation, Drs. Howard Frank and Paul Zoll implanted a long-term Electrodyne pacemaker. Two years later the same patient was admitted with a fractured electrode, causing a disconnect between the pacemaker and the heart, which by default left the patient vulnerable. Once again, during a pastoral visit by the same priest, the patient suffered another cardiac fibrillation arrest. Whether by design, or merely coincidence, the déjà vu sequence of events repeated, including revival and survival. It might be said that a guardian angel in priestly habit looked over that man's shoulder.[39]

Many early pioneers in medical electronics were based at a medical center or collaborated with physicians conducting experiments in the field. Albert Morris is an anomaly. He was not affiliated with a medical center and he did not have a continuous collaborative relationship with a physician investigator. Albert was an independent electrical engineer and an entrepreneur who claims priority for designing and manufacturing the first production model open-chest defibrillator, for designing and introducing the first transthoracic pacemaker into clinical practice, and for designing and producing the first transthoracic defibrillator for use in man.[40] His later claims about a transthoracic pacemaker and defibrillator are difficult to substantiate. As a result, they created tension between Albert Morris on America's west coast and Paul Zoll on the east coast.

ELEVEN

ALBERT MORRIS: A PIONEER WHO DESERVES GREATER RECOGNITION

Albert Morris had several distinguished careers. Medical electronics was the earliest and most memorable in the private sector. Albert was the first to manufacture an open-chest defibrillator and believes that he was the first to produce a closed-chest pacemaker and defibrillator in the Western Hemisphere. Such claims put him in direct contention with Paul Zoll over primacy as developer of closed-chest devices.

Albert was born, raised, and remained in the Bronx, New York, until completing high school in 1935. He relocated to California in search of adventure and an affordable higher education. At the University of California, Los Angeles, mechanical and electrical engineering were his consuming favorite subjects. The last year of undergraduate college study was spent at The University of California, Berkeley, where he shared a portion of an off-campus rooming house with his cousin Milton Waldman, a pre-medical student.

On December 7, 1941 – the "day that shall live in infamy," when Franklin Delano Roosevelt announced that the nation was at war – Albert immediately visited a naval recruiting station. But poor eye sight torpedoed his enlistment plans. Self-discipline, determination, coaching from an optometrist, and total recall of a memorized standard eye chart were rewarded with a certified *pass* on the visual examination in February 1943. Morris received a commission as ensign in the U.S. Navy and orders to attend specialty school at the Massachusetts Institute of Technology and several other universities that speedily trained Albert in radar, guidance, and other tracking systems. He became the electronics officer on the USS Solomons aircraft carrier, which patrolled for submarines between the coasts of South America and Africa. Albert's responsibility was "… to make things work with very high reliability."[1] After 18 months of sea duty, he spent the remainder of active military service at the Airborne Coordinating Group of the Naval Research Laboratory, and a few months on temporary duty in San Francisco. When released back to civilian life at war's end, Morris became the first civilian employee of the Scientific Branch of the Office of Naval Research (ONR), an organization that awarded grants to industrial institutions, colleges and universities. During a seven-year tenure, from 1946 to 1952, Morris reviewed all electronic and related engineering scientific research activities. The ONR also allowed him to attend graduate school and to directly participate in some of the research projects that the agency supported.

A fateful conversation in 1949 redirected Albert's destiny. Cousin Milton Waldman, now an anesthesiologist M.D., asked Albert to build an open-chest defibrillator for Frank Gerbode, a visiting thoracic surgeon at San Francisco's Veterans Hospital at Fort Miley. The request followed Claude Beck's successful first known open-chest defibrillation in 1947, which had generated enormous interest among his colleagues, including Frank Gerbode, who would go on to became a leading heart surgeon on the local and national scene. In 1949, Gerbode was the first doctor at the San Francisco Veteran's Hospital to request that a defibrillator be made to his specifications.[2,3] After Morris built and delivered the first unit, he received several more orders from Fort Miley.

Those early defibrillators were made from donated surplus parts gleaned at Stanford University Laboratories. The paddles were fabricated from stainless steel cooking spatulas purchased at a local five-and-dime store.[4] Sensing an opportunity to satisfy a growing demand, Albert became the first commercial manufacturer of clinical open- chest cardiac defibrillators. Marketing the machines as the Morris Clinical Defibrillator, he preceded one competitor by six months and another by one year.[5] Throughout his life, Morris made a distinction between the concepts of *inventing* and *creating* by maintaining that he never invented his defibrillator or pacemaker, although they were of his own design and were created from basic principles of engineering, electrical theory and an extensive search of the literature. If the company had a mission statement it might have been "To widely disseminate and make available life-saving cardiac equipment."[6]

Albert Morris the entrepreneur was unlike his contemporaries involved in creating electrocardiac therapies. William Kouwenhoven developed both the science and its application at Johns Hopkins. Claude Beck became familiar with the science developed by his colleague, Carl Wiggers, at Western Reserve University and had an open chest defibrillator built with the help of James Rand, of the Rand Development Corporation.[7,8] Albert Morris did it on his own, without a direct link to a hospital or research organization. Between 1949 and 1952, he traveled the 11 western states by day to view research facilities that sought or had ONR grants. By night, Albert introduced his defibrillator to hospitals, emphasizing the importance of being up to date in cardiac resuscitation. In 1952, his ONR territory expanded to include the remaining 37 states. A committed missionary, he spread "the word" that proper resuscitation foiled death..

Morris, long on ideas and short on time, juggled three commitments. In addition to expanding his defibrillator business and being productive in his job at ONR, Morris had married in 1943 and was raising a family. What's more, he supervised production of his equipment at an independent firm's "factory", which was really a private garage.[9] Early purchasers of the defibrillator included such notables as heart surgeon Walton Lillehei and the eminent William Kouwenhoven. Driven by prospects of a growing enterprise, Albert resigned from ONR to nurture his business, which had been in need of a growth spurt from an expanded product line. Morris accomplished that mission by joining forces with Elliot Levinthal of Levinthal Electronic Products. After the 1953 merger, the Morris Defibrillator Company remained intact as a defined division within Levinthal. All medical devices were now manufactured in-house by Leventhal. A new Morris Clinical Closed Chest Pacemaker was introduced in 1953, the same year as the merger.

The marketing of this closed-chest pacemaker caused a skirmish between Albert Morris and Paul Zoll. The new Morris pacemaker was competitive with its Electrodyne counterpart in size and price. Albert believed that each performed well, but that his had superior engineering.[10] He also believed that

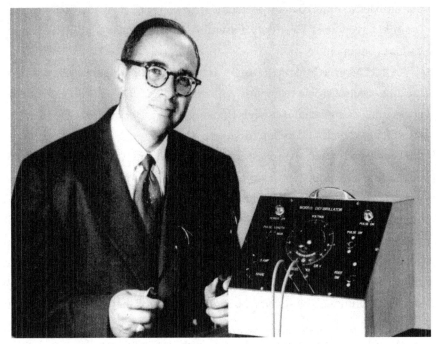

Albert Morris with his Morris internal defibrillator. He is holding the paddles. When in use, they were placed on the surface of the heart. Courtesy of Albert Morris. With permission.

his was the first production-model closed-chest pacemaker made, setting up a conflict with Zoll over that distinction.

Morris had intimate personal knowledge of his pacemaker's performance, going back to its inception, when he tested it on himself. The Morris pacemaker also underwent a limited animal test trial in the San Francisco Cardiovascular Research Laboratory of Dr. Sanford Leeds. The most extensive pre-market trial, however, was near fatal self-testing. "Since I did not have an animal laboratory to work with, I did all the experiments on myself," he explained.[11] On one occasion, curious to learn how fast he could pace- race his heart, Albert tried and passed out. Fortunately, the pacing electrodes broke away from his chest during the unexpected descent to the cement floor. If the electrodes had remained in place, Albert most likely would have been added to the list of investigator self-test deaths. The list includes George Mines, an advocate of self-testing, who in 1914 was found unconscious in his laboratory still attached to experimental physiological equipment. Mines died later that day. An autopsy failed to find a cause, which led to speculation that self-testing resulted in a self-induced fatal arrhythmia.[12,13] Some colleagues believed that Mines might have been observing the vulnerable period of his cardiac cycle with electrical stimuli, a concept that he had introduced in an animal model. While reflecting on his own brush with death, Morris opined, "Part of life is to live up to your stupidity."[14]

Tom Corbin, an assistant to Albert in the development of the transthoracic pacer and defibrillator, explained that collaborating with a physician investigator to develop and clinically test an instrument is tantamount to forcing an endorsement of the device by a spokesperson of the medical establishment.[15] Morris would eventually turn over the entire medical instrument unit to his assistant engineers, Corbin and Elliot Farnsworth.

Self-testing mishaps weren't the only hazards that confronted pioneers in electrocardic therapy. Several medical electronic pioneers suffered inadvertent electrical shocks or near electrocution in the course of their work. Among them were William Kouwenhoven[16] and Earl Bakken[17] – a founder of the device maker Medtronic Incorporated. Albert Morris avoided similar jolts while working, but suffered two electric shocks while enjoying some leisure moments at his home. The first severe jolt occurred while in his swimming pool. The Pacific Gas and Electric Company "diagnosed" a wiring problem that required a costly fix. About a year later, Albert received another shock while in the pool. The electrical company's erroneous diagnosis might have resulted in Morris' death if the second shock had been more severe. A friend who was a senior scientist at Medtronic properly diagnosed and corrected an electrical grounding problem after his testing equipment proved that activating the kitchen toaster would simultaneously heat bread and shock a swimmer in the pool.[18]

Albert Morris has no memory of instrument failures, but has a clear memory of receiving an accusatory phone call from Paul Zoll related to pacemaker patent infringement. The call must have been more of a scare tactic than a threat because by edict of Harvard Medical School, Electrodyne held no patents on its devices. What's more, in the absence of an explanation, the Electrodyne closed-chest pacemaker may not have even qualified for a patent because it was described in a sole early publication as "a modification of existing physiological stimulators."[19] Years later, Alan Belgard explained that he modified the wave forms of his own long-standing Electrodyne stimulators that were intended for nerve and muscle measurements.[20] Yet both Albert Morris and Alan Belgard maintain that they solely created their instruments from basic electronic principles and from data in the published literature. In any event, the threat from Zoll did not seem to alarm Morris, who was Bronx born and Bronx bred. He described his reaction, "I told Zoll to go to hell."[21,22]

It seems that Zoll's out-of-character bluff was triggered by his belief that Morris had copied the Electrodyne design. Much of that belief seems to stem from the close timing between the releases of the two products. "We did everything we knew and picked out the best and they (Morris) built a pacemaker," Zoll said when relating his views years later. He continued to rail against Morris, "Within a month of Electrodyne putting the pacer on the market there was a competitor in California without the two or three years that they (Zoll, Belgard, et al) had spent in the laboratory." [23]

In publications, Albert Morris appears to agree in general that "his pacer and the competition (Electrodyne) got started about the same time."[24] More clarification about the timing of the devices came during a 1988 legal proceeding. A law firm, defending the Physio-Control company in a patent infringement claim brought by ZMI (Zoll) Corporation, asked Albert Morris to help its cause by providing data about his pacemaker and electrodes. Morris welcomed the request, eagerly cooperated and was thankful for the opportunity to retaliate against a person he considered to be a false accuser whose behavior Morris characterized as "belligerent, unpleasant and inaccurate."[25]

During the 1988 legal proceedings, Zoll acknowledged that the Morris closed-chest pacemaker was available in 1953, saying "I heard that the new instrument, the Morris instrument, had come out within a few months of the first ones that the Electrodyne people had sold and it looked a little different, but it was identical in function. … it was very competitive with Electrodyne."[26]

Other evidence suggests that Zoll felt rancor about the Morris device. Paul Zoll received a letter from Elliot Levinthal in early 1955 with a testimonial from an anesthesiologist about a successful patient outcome resulting from prompt application of a Morris Clinical Pacemaker in the operating room. Zoll wrote to the source requesting detailed patient data and consent to include the case in a manuscript about paced patients with successful outcomes.[27] The case never appeared in the final article that contained 25 cases gathered from six Massachusetts hospitals. All patients mentioned were managed with an Electrodyne pacemaker. The Morris Clinical Pacemaker case might have been excluded because consent to publish was not granted, a deadline passed or the case was deleted by design.[28]

What about Morris' claim of primacy over Zoll for developing the first closed-chest defibrillator specifically intended for human use? Proof of successful human application is one way to substantiate that claim. Here Morris made an interesting case that lacks conclusive evidence.

While traveling about the country promoting his open chest defibrillator in 1954, Morris met the head of the Aero Medical Laboratory at Wright-Patterson Air Force Base in Ohio. Volunteers were undergoing tests to quantify their physiological stress limits. Those who passed would be qualified to pilot earth-orbiting spacecraft. To test for gravitational force stress (G-force), researchers spun a pilot in a centrifuge at the end of a 50-foot boom. If a cardiac arrest were to occur during the study, there was not enough time to slow down the centrifuge, remove the anti G-force suit and save the pilot in a race against death. Morris was asked, "Can you build a transthoracic defibrillator-pacemaker that will remotely activate to defibrillate or pace a test pilot through pre-positioned electrodes?" Morris boldly accepted the challenge without knowledge of it ever being done before. He then inquired, why the need for this type of apparatus? The answer was so vague that, as Morris later revealed "I have always suspected that they lost one or more bright men in their early tests and there was no way the government would publicize this ..."[29] Morris received a purchase order from the laboratory in 1954.

Both Albert Morris and colleague Tom Corbin concur that the defibrillator/pacer was built to Air Force specifications as a production model and delivered sometime in 1955. Unfortunately, they do not know any details regarding its use or effectiveness. Many elements of the space program were conducted in secret and were likely classified as such.[30]

Shortly after delivery of the Wright-Patterson defibrillator, Morris received an order for two more from Litton Industries, Los Angeles, California, which had a contract with the Naval Research Laboratory space program test facility at Moffet Field Naval Air Station in Mountain View and Sunnyvale, California.

At Moffet, the Navy also was attempting to learn if humans had the capacity to explore outer space. Tom Corbin echoed Albert Morris' account of the test site and the concerns of its scientists. "Their concept was that if the G-force got high enough to send the heart into fibrillation, the experimenter could deliver a shock immediately instead of losing precious time waiting for the centrifuge to slow down and stop."[31] Corbin described these vanishing defibrillators as large, too heavy for one person to carry, capable of delivering 1,000 volts, operating on line voltage and basically a "laboratory curiosity."[32]

Apparently the three archival defibrillators delivered to the test facilities have vanished and there has been no public review of their use or effectiveness. The Aero Medical Laboratory published one review of human tolerance to centrifuge velocity of acceleration (G-force),[33] and the same facility published a separate, later study.[34] The authors described several induced cardiovascular problems such as rapid heart rate, low blood pressure, chest pain, presumed low cardiac output and blackout with temporary unconscious status. Neither study made mention of life threatening arrhythmias. One must conclude that the Morris Closed Chest Clinical Defibrillator-Pacemaker's contribution to the Air Force and Navy space programs remains unknown or at best shrouded in government secrecy. Moreover, detailed corporate records to substantiate purchase orders and delivery dates have been lost, reinforcing the adage that ground-breaking investigators must compulsively document their findings to receive proper attribution for their discoveries.

Paul Zoll succeeded in closed-chest defibrillating his first patient in 1955, the same year that Morris delivered his first production-model closed-chest defibrillator to the Aero Medical Laboratory. But Zoll published his results in 1956. William Kouwenhoven followed with his first human success in 1957.[35] When Johns Hopkins stopped making Kouwenhoven defibrillators for other hospitals in their on-site electrical shop, Kouwenhoven's direct-current defibrillator concepts were merged into production models manufactured by Corbin-Farnsworth Incorporated[36], which was the third iteration of the original Morris defibrillator venture after Corbin-Farnsworth acquired the Morris Defibrillator division from Leventhal Electronic Products.

Albert Morris was the first to manufacture an open-chest defibrillator for the general medical community, and he might have been the first in the Western

Hemisphere to produce a closed-chest defibrillator for human use. Regrettably, after delivery to the space program, his work went off the radar. The closed-chest commercial Morris Clinical Pacemaker appeared after Paul Zoll's initial human successes with a borrowed Grass stimulator and all hard evidence indicates that it trailed the Electrodyne production model by a brief interval.

Still, Albert Morris is a pioneer deserving of greater recognition. What is his place in the history of electrocardiac therapy? He answered the question when he summarized his experience: "I am most proud of my contributions in the medical electronics field. I believe that I have been one of the pioneers in the application of cardiac resuscitation and monitoring in surgery."[37]

TWELVE

A TALE OF TWO PEOPLE: THE PHYSICIAN/SCIENTIST AND THE RECREATIONALIST

Paul Zoll's demeanor in the workplace was in stark contrast to the behavior he displayed while relaxed at play in his backyard, where his recreation seemed almost detached from medical responsibilities. Almost. In tune with the times, Paul was a solo practitioner committed to an "on call" lifestyle while serving as a family doctor, internist and cardiologist. What's more, he welcomed critical problems that arose in the course of patient care because they catalyzed his research. He seldom took a vacation and he accepted the unending distractions created by demands from, or about, acutely ill patients whether he was in the research lab or at home after hours.[1] In the laboratory, he was generally serious and goal oriented, shedding his white, stiffly starched doctor cloak at the door and crossing its threshold to problem-solve among equals. But when treating patients or teaching at the hospital, Paul was known to be autocratic and stern. He demanded a lot from himself and expected no less from others.[2] At Beth Israel Hospital he was among a group of most knowledgeable physicians who were assigned supervisory responsibility for patients on the teaching wards. That meant he was responsible for teams of medical students and post-graduate trainees. Paul was authoritarian in establishing his diagnostic and therapeutic plans for patients. He entertained alternative ideas from trainees, but rarely deviated from his prescribed course. Students were in awe of Paul's lightning fast mind. Yet his reluctance to relinquish control, to alter his diagnostic or therapeutic plan, or to delegate even minor decisions that might modify a patient's outcome were a cumulative source of irritation to qualified trainees on the cusp of graduating to positions of authority. One group vented its displeasure during an irreverent theatrical production that was an annual tradition at commencement time. During the event, a performer asked the rhetorical question, "What is a Zoll?" Another answered, "It is a prominent physician and a unit of resistance!"[3]

Another tradition was for each teaching physician to entertain his or her cadre of pupils at the conclusion of a course. Trainees who attended a yard party at Paul's home described him as an uninhibited "wild man" diving and stroking briskly about the swimming pool.[4] In contrast to the trainees' often intimidating experiences at the hospital, a great time was had by all.

They witnessed the recreational side of Paul Zoll that he did not display in his professional roles as researcher and physician. The only place Paul appeared to truly relax was in the recreational space he created at his home in Newton, a suburb of Boston. The driveway sloped down the right side of the house, then turned sharply behind the building where a powerful outboard motor was tilted on the stern of a boat that Paul trailered with his shopworn automobile to water ski at nearby Lake Cochichuate.[5] A swimming pool, utility shed and tennis court were compactly arranged within the fenced property behind the house. The yard was the family's chosen place to relax alone or with relatives, friends, patients that became friends, and colleagues who Paul selectively limited in number.[6,7] Janet very seldom entertained within the home since Paul and she preferred the yard. Daughter Mary recalled that Dr. Mark Altshule was the only person in memory that Janet ever had for a formal dinner, saying "She actually cooked a meal and invited someone over. Janet put on a real show. She never invited anyone else."[8]

Paul's center of gravity would not permit his home to be a sanctuary for rest alone. Even while relaxing on the tennis court or at poolside, Paul could not forsake his doctoring. That is where he spotted cousin David's melanoma.[9] Paul stayed in touch with his medical practice by a telephone on a long cord that reached from the house to the swimming pool or the near end of the tennis court beyond. He was rarely off-call.

What's more, Paul did evening and nighttime work at home the year round. That included the seven months that seasonal weather in New England allowed comfortable outdoor recreation, and also seasons when seeking refuge in the yard was not an option. After the family's dinner, the kitchen table was often transformed into a platform to birth medical manuscripts. When Arthur Linenthal and Paul first started crafting their publications in the Zoll kitchen, they worked on a wooden table with coarse grain that resembled the peaks and valleys of a range of hills. Paul and Arthur wrote on clipboards to prevent pen or pencil from puncturing the paper on the grooved tabletop. A new table with a Formica surface solved the problem.[10]

Paul and Arthur were precise writers who strove for perfection. They argued about context, punctuation and grammar. On more than one occasion, Arthur returned home exhausted from a session the pair deemed successful. In one case, he told his wife that they "…made progress tonight. We wrote a sentence and accepted it."[11]

Paul did not watch television nor listen to music. He had no interest in spectator sports and he summed up his attitude about them when he encouraged his children to participate rather than observe. Paul was a participant and an above-average athlete. When a youth, he could sink a basket from half court,[12] and played touch football after school – an activity that he later continued as a young doctor during lunchtime with research personnel at the Beth Israel Hospital parking lot.[13] At home he enjoyed tennis and became a competent swimmer – yard activities that Paul understandably selected because, unlike team sports, they did not require much commitment or planning and could be interrupted and resumed at will.

Paul's love of tennis carried over from his boyhood, when he had learned the game on the courts at Franklin Field. As an adult, Paul often played on his home court by the waning light of weekday summer evenings or after lunch on weekends. By necessity, the rules were bent. During the entirety of so-called exercise or a game, Paul remained close to the telephone on the near-side of the court, because of intermittent calls from doctors or patients. That meant that the sun, past its apex on its daily westerly journey, always faced Paul's opponent so that his serves and returns had the glare as an ally. Even without that advantage, "Paul was fast, tenacious and showed little mercy in dispatching opponents, including awestruck doctors in training,"[14] according to one observer. On a hot day, after the last point, Paul might pause in the shadow of a tall courtside hemlock tree that edged the property, masking perspiration that ran down his face and bare chest. The shadow also masked Paul's codified apparel of faded bathing suit and tattered sneakers. Emerging from the shadows, his silhouette often raced to the pool and jumped into its cooling water.[15]

Born an unnatural swimmer, Paul did not acquire the skill in his youth, although, like most Bostonians, he went to the beach in the heat of summer to catch an ocean breeze and wade in the cool surf. In his final term at Harvard College in 1936, in order to finalize his high academic achievement and have *summa cum laude* inscribed on his graduation diploma, Paul was required to pass a swimming test. In fact, if he failed the test, according to an unconfirmed, likely apocryphal myth, the penalty would be a certificate of attendance rather than a sheepskin parchment.

Two version of Paul's performance during the swimming test have been reported. The first is that he succeeded, but nearly drowned.[16] The second is that he nearly drowned while failing, but was given a "pass" by a kindly instructor after Paul made a solemn pledge to improve with practice.[17] He eventually became a good swimmer and an accomplished water skier. The Harvard College promise may have contributed to those abilities, but a traumatic incident certainly encouraged Zoll to acquire aquatic skills. It occurred soon after the war, when Janet and Paul spent their vacation working

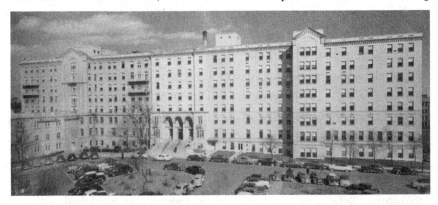

The asphalt and lawns bordering the parking areas at the front entrance of the Beth Israel Hospital (Circa 1940–1950) were used for recreational touch–football games by the trainees and staff members during lunch break. Courtesy of the Ruth and David Freiman Archives at Beth Israel Deaconess Medical Center. With permission.

as nurse and physician at a children's camp. While there, a youngster died from accidental drowning. Years later, the Zolls prohibited their own children from attending summer camp until they became proficient swimmers. Accordingly, the children took instruction at nearby Crystal Lake. Paul also took advanced swimming instruction there to support a growing interest in safe boating and water skiing.[18]

Regarding his children, Paul commented in his Harvard College 25th class reunion report, "There was time however to get married and in 1947 to have a tremendous good fortune to acquire a pair of assorted twins who have managed to keep me hopping since then with the excitement, joy, pride, dismay, anguish and the end of boredom forever." The entry is his most powerful revelation of joy in family and pleasure in fatherhood. The reason for dismay is unclear. The anguish might have been the circumstances of Janet's pregnancy and delivery. When she suspected the possibility of carrying twins, the obstetrician disagreed, saying, "Yes, there is one in your belly and one in your imagination." But Janet, an experienced nurse, was certain that she heard two fetal hearts while listening through a stethoscope placed on her belly. Paul confirmed the finding. The pregnancy was difficult and did not carry to term. Ross preceded Mary by minutes. The seven-month preemies required extended intensive nursing care. Ross was discharged first to Janet's full-time care at home. Mary remained in the hospital for weeks, with Paul visiting her each evening en route from work to home.[19]

Raising the children brought a combination of pleasures and challenges, with rewards ultimately realized. If tennis with a guest opponent concluded early, Paul might stay on the court and play a game with Mary – her brother, Ross, never mastered its fundamentals enough to participate. Paul often frolicked with Ross and Mary in the pool or brought the children water skiing. Probably the biggest challenge occurred when Mary, as a teenager, endured a head-first collision into a tree while sledding. She was unconscious for several days, then suffered severe headaches and a prolonged post-concussive syndrome. For two years, inability to concentrate kept her from school. Paul and Janet could do no more than hope for improvement, and then hope for further recovery after Mary progressed enough to perform literature searches to support Dr. Mark Altshule's research projects. Over time, as Mary's recovery continued, the Zolls' anxiety yielded to mere concern and then to complete relief. Mary not only returned to high school, she was the class valedictorian at graduation. Mary next moved onto Vassar College and then graduate school to earn a doctorate in biochemistry, followed by teaching appointments at Northeastern University and Massachusetts Institute of Technology.

Ross, in his father's footsteps, attended Harvard College and then earned a graduate degree in physics at the University of Chicago. He pursued research in that field before returning to Boston to help Paul solve problems in medical electronics and arrhythmia management. Ross then entered a unique accelerated program leading to a medical degree at the University of Miami. As of 2013, he is a practicing anesthesiologist with hobbies that include raising dogs and piloting a plane. The achievements of the twins prove that Paul and Janet's pride in their children was always justified.

Characterizing Paul Zoll can appear like a tale of two people because his behaviors were so different. His body and soul were totally committed to stressful academic pursuits in his workplace and were totally committed to non-stressful pursuits in his recreational space. Yet he appeared to be totally comfortable in the two primary places he created with his lifestyle. He seemed at ease, as if on holiday, in his recreational space at home, to the point that at times his associates could describe him as uninhibited. On weekends, he went to the hospital each morning, even though no patient had to be seen, because he believed that there was no end to his medical mission.[20]

According to some accounts, when Paul was at the homes of close friends, most times it was "painful" to engage him in conversation because he was preoccupied and consumed with his hospital or research work. He often went off and sat in a corner.[21] In most social settings and situations outside of his personal recreational spaces, Paul was known to be shy, ill at ease, and a man of few words. In a letter, Paul acknowledged the shyness he felt during the very start of his internship at Beth Israel Hospital. He described how the medical resident "…insisted on introducing me to the chief nurses on all the floors; worse than that, he made me present each of them with a flower. This event produced severe social embarrassment that I still remember vividly."[22]

According to one friend, "There was nobody who talked as little and was so small and yet took up so much space. He was a little guy. He never said anything. He just filled the room. If you didn't speak to him he wouldn't say anything and if you did, complete silence might follow."[23] Another observer noted that "Paul didn't mingle, didn't care to mingle. He answered questions in monosyllables."[24] Rather than anti-social, Paul appeared to be simply not in-terested in the small

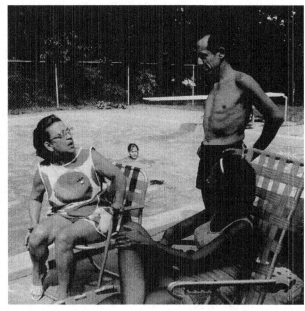

Paul and Janet Zoll in conversation at pool side in their back yard. The identity of the other persons is unknown. The tennis court is not in view. Courtesy of Maggie Frank O'Connor. With permission.

talk and chatter that prevails at most social events. He often opined that "people died from smoking too much, eating too much, drinking too much and talking too much."[25,26]

Although he was normally very quiet, Paul's speech was not guided or influenced by political correctness. He was honest in academic affairs and in personal relationships.[27] When asked to pass judgment on a physician colleague who was recommended to perform a consultation, Paul answered, "He thinks he is good… but I have my doubts."[28]

On occasion, Paul initiated a conversation that seemed to need a pretense to get started. The wife of his next-door neighbor, whose husband had been a B-17 bomber pilot during World War II, explained that Paul sometimes started with a masked technical question that related to his unpublished research. But that wasn't always the case. He most often was compassionate and exchanged formalities and pleasantries of the day. Once, while on the neighbor's porch, Paul noticed that their pet spaniel, Buffer, lay whining and lethargic. After a hurried examination, Paul rushed away and returned with a stethoscope and a black medical bag. When the excited doctor-turned-veterinarian re-examined the dog, he exclaimed "atrial fibrillation is the problem!" Zoll opened the black bag, searched for a bottle, administered a tablet of digitalis, and left instructions to bring the dog to his office the next day. There he found that normal heart rhythm had returned. It was maintained for years with daily digitalis.[29]

Paul's common disregard for social standards also showed in his personal style and appearance. Paul was the most unaffected person that cousin Elliot Mahler ever met. He had simple tastes and "…just didn't care about his appearance." He didn't dress in fashionable clothes,[30] which was obvious to all. A longtime patient noted that "He was shabbily attired, but it did not concern him. His shirt was worn and would have embarrassed most men, but not Dr. Zoll . . . he made many house calls in a beat up old car that questionably could make it up our driveway. In appreciation for his many house calls and kindness, I sent him two conservative silk ties from a fancy men's store–after receiving them, his wife called to acknowledge the gifts, adding that Paul would probably never wear them."[31] On another occasion, Paul did accept a gift tie. He would not accept payment for services after treating a student nurse who had pneumonia. So she knitted the tie for him. He wore it every day for a month until the nurse told him to change to another.[32]

Although Zoll was quiet and kept to himself, nothing suggests that he was aloof, haughty, or held himself above other people. Just the opposite. Humility and the absence of self promotion were defining characteristics of Paul Zoll.

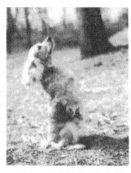

Buffer, a neighbor's dog, appears healthy and happy after Paul Zoll's diagnosis and treatment of atrial fibrillation. Courtesy of Daphne Glassman. With permission.

When congratulated for a medical discovery, he often attributed success to coworkers. Similarly, when he received official, personal honors or recognition, he seemed to accept them as a surrogate for the discoveries that he helped to uncover.

In one case, Zoll received a letter from a physician in Calcutta, India, who wished to inspire children on a path towards science and medicine by writing monographs about transforming achievements in those fields. The physician-educator mentioned that he had written about Edward Jenner, Alexander Fleming, Madam Curie and Louis Pasteur, among others. He now wanted to write about Paul Zoll and his discoveries. Paul replied that he "…thought it absurd to be put in the company of Jenner, Pasteur, etcetera" and that he would cooperate only if the author could not be dissuaded.[33] On another occasion, Paul received a letter of introduction and a completed form from an eminent professor nominating him for a prestigious American Heart Association award. Paul was asked to review the application for accuracy prior to submission. He expressed his surprise at being worthy of consideration and his thanks for an opportunity to review the document, which he returned

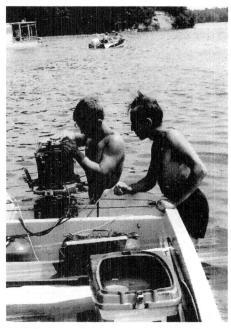

As Paul looks on, Ross Zoll repairs the outboard motor that interrupted their plans to water ski at Lake Cochichuate. Courtesy of Maggie Frank O'Connor. With permission.

with edits that corrected only spelling and grammatical errors.[34] Others might have returned the papers without the editing, but with additional information and references meant to increase their chances of receiving the award.

Alan Belgard, Ross Zoll and Leona Norman Zarsky offered insightful explanations for the contrasting perceptions of Paul Zoll. Alan, "At the lake or playing tennis, he was a different guy than his interactions in the hospital … It was almost as if he could throw a switch."[35] Ross, "He had a rough demeanor when necessary, but it was totally an act."[36] Leona, "He had a lot of feelings for his sick patients that he had to cover up, otherwise, he would have broken down … He was soft inside. I saw the soft side…"[37] Zarsky concluded that the leader among equals in the lab and the recreationalist at play, "…was funny, fun and supportive – not the image seen by the general public."[38]

THIRTEEN

AMONG THE LEADERS IN THE RACE TO IMPLANT A LONG-TERM PACEMAKER

The cast of characters in the long-term implantable pacemaker story includes scientists and engineers pushing the limits of technology, courageous doctors exploring the unknown, and desperate patients. (See table on next page.)

The technical barrier they all faced was to shrink a pacemaker, including its energy source and all components, into a small container suitable for implantation under the skin. Additionally, the pacer's wire electrode(s) that completed the system had to provide a durable internal bridge from the heart to the pacemaker. The race for primacy was an international competition that harnessed creativity and available technology. Although most of the major advances occurred in Scandinavia and the northeastern United States, contributions also came from determined workers in Europe, South America and Canada.

Åke Senning and Rune Elmqvist
Sweden

In 1958, Arne Larsson, a 43-year-old Swedish engineer, became the first to receive a partially contained long-term implanted pacemaker. Like all of the early pacemaker implant patients, he suffered life-threatening Stokes-Adams attacks.[1] Arne's wife, Else Marie, read in an American magazine that a human

Pacemaker Pioneers and Patients

IMPLANT TEAM	PLACE AND DATE	PACEMAKER	PATIENT	EARLY OUTCOME
Äke Senning Rune Elmqvist	Sweden Oct. 10, 1958 Oct. 11, 1958	Rechargeable Made in-house	Arne Larsson	Failed in 6 hours Failed within 6 weeks
William Glenn Alexander Mauro	New Haven, Conn. USA Jan. 29, 1959	Radiofrequency Made in-house	William Tobbler	Failed on day 20
William Chardack Wilson Greatbatch	Buffalo, N.Y. USA Lead implant Stage 1 April 18, 1960 Pacer implant Stage 2 June 6, 1960	Self-contained Made by Wilson Greatbatch	Frank Henefelt	Stage 1 Uncomplicated Stage 2 Uncomplicated
Paul Zoll Alan Belgard Howard Frank	Boston, Mass. USA Lead implant Stage 1 July 20, 1960 Pacer implant Stage 2 Oct. 28, 1960	Self-contained Made by Electrodyne	Michael Seiffer	Stage 1 Uncomplicated Stage 2 Erosion Infection Pacer exteriorized
Adrian Kantrowitz	Brooklyn, N.Y. USA March 22, 1961	Self-contained Rate adjustable Made by General Electric	Rose Cohen	Uncomplicated

heart had been successfully stimulated with a battery-powered pacemaker. When she raised the issue with Dr. Äke Senning at the Karolinska Institute, near Stockholm, she learned that experiments were being conducted on dogs with heart wires drawn through their skin that connected to an external pacemaker. But Senning was against the method in humans because it was an invitation for an inevitable infection. Nonetheless, with Else's encouragement, her husband volunteered to accept any type of pacemaker procedure because he failed to improve after numerous drugs trials, and death appeared certain in the absence of a miracle. Thus Plato's aphorism, "necessity is the mother of invention" put fire to the feet of surgeon Äke Senning and physician Rune Elmqvist, who was also a self-taught engineer. They immediately began work on an implantable system. Else's daily requests for progress reports and her unrestrained hopes for success drove them on at breakneck speed. It was an extraordinary example of a new initiative focusing on a solitary patient. By the time Elmqvist cobbled together some pacemakers for abbreviated tests in dogs and built two prototypes for his patient, Arne was in such critical circumstances that he needed resuscitation 30 times on some days. Elmqvist encased the components of the pacemaker in epoxy resin potted in a Kiwi shoe polish can. The prototype unit's batteries required recharging from an induction coil attached to an external unit. Six hours after insertion, Arne's initial pacer failed. The next day his doctors replaced it with the backup unit that also developed immediate problems. It completely failed to pace within six weeks.[2]

Stokes-Adams disease is unpredictable with life expectancy of two years from onset to death. The Gods smiled upon Arne Larsson. Remarkably, after his second prototype unit failed, his untreated complete heart block and continuous slow heart rate stabilized *without* a working electronic pacemaker. Larsson suffered only infrequent, minor Stokes-Adams attacks between mid December 1958 and November 1961 when his doctors implanted a fully contained, self-sustaining, reliable pacemaker.[3] The three-year non-paced hiatus was unconditionally ignored in a statement by the third-generation manufacturer of the original Elmqvist and Elema Shonander pacemakers, the commercial units that grew out of Elmqvist's pioneering work on Larsson's behalf. Instead, the company claimed that Larsson had not endured a syncopal attack nor cardiac rhythm disturbance since his first pacemaker placement in 1958.[4]

The long thread of Arne's charmed life thinned over time and finally broke in 2002 when he died. He was named in The Guinness Book of Records for having 26 pacemaker implants between 1958 and 1996. A perfected model of the Elmqvist-Elema Shonander rechargeable pacemaker was implanted in several isolated European and South American patients between 1958 and 1960.[5,6]

Paul Zoll and Alan Belgard
Preliminary Efforts
Boston, Massachusetts, USA

Paul Zoll had been on a quest to eliminate fear of unpredictable faints, the associated need for football helmets to protect skulls and brains during falls and ultimately to provide security against sudden death. That quest started prior to the day that Mr. A, known as the first externally paced patient, returned home without prospects for long-term cardiac stability. Paul Zoll and Alan Belgard knew that their victory was shallow and believed that they had a moral imperative to build a long-term pacemaker.[7]

They conducted their first animal experiments in 1955, using heart wires drawn out of the abdomen to an external pacemaker.[8] Progress was slow. In their next step they tested radiofrequency pacing systems consisting of implanted receivers that captured signals broadcast from external vacuum-tube transmitters that were initially powered from a wall outlet, then by a huge battery. The arrival of transistor technology enabled engineers to create small battery-powered radiofrequency transmitters. Transistors were also the crucial element to building totally implantable, fully contained pacemakers. Another barrier was creating reliable electrodes to connect from the pacemaker to the heart. In 1960, after five long years of trial and tribulation to develop an acceptable pacemaker electrode lead, Zoll, Belgard and Electrodyne were able to proceed with their plan to place a fully implantable self-contained pacemaker in a human.[9]

At the time, all workers in the field expected their implanted pacer units to perform below specifications. They accepted nickel cadmium rechargeable batteries and mercury zinc batteries that were projected to last approximately four years, but failed in two. They accepted pacers potted in epoxy resin that permitted both hydrogen gas to escape and body fluids to enter – potentially short circuiting a unit with moisture. Some investigators accepted the unacceptable rate of electrode failure that stifled Zoll's progress. For many years investigators seemed unable to solve the problems of electrode breakage and unremitting electrode-mediated escalation of the energy required to stimulate the heart. Too often, the energy required to pace exceeded the output of the pacemaker. Scar formation at the interface between the electrode and heart muscle caused the problem. Following a series of wire electrode fractures, Paul recorded a frustrating, yet humorous dead-end experience. Engineers at the Massachusetts Institute of Technology had referred Paul to the Simplex Wire Company to find an acceptable electrode. After estimating the small amount of wire he would need, Paul learned that Simplex only supplied minimum quantities of the wire in very large lots the size of railroad boxcars. When asked to describe the needed specifications and properties, Paul requested a flexion tolerance of more than 36 million flexes per year for 50 years, which approximated the lifelong needs of a young adult. He learned that Simplex could provide wire with a flexion tolerance of only several thousand before fracture.[10] So Paul continued to experiment with a variety of electrodes with different metals, coatings, insulations and configurations in hundreds of animals.[11]

Zoll only had confidence in his own findings. He did not trust discoveries "from elsewhere." His skepticism, once entrenched, was almost impossible to overcome. After being long stymied by electrode failures, he accepted help from General Electric. His intermediary with the company was a patient who was employed as a scientist by General Electric and who offered Paul advice on methods to improve pacemaker electrode longevity and overall performance.[12] In an extraordinary gesture, General Electric supplied its own prototypes and exchanged information with Zoll in compliance with its public service policy, even though the company was simultaneously partnering with Adrian Kantrowitz at Maimonides Hospital in Brooklyn, New York, to develop and manufacture its own version of a fully implantable pacemaker.

While Zoll struggled to overcome electrode fracture and threshold problems, surgeon Samuel Hunter and engineer Norman Roth in Minneapolis, Minnesota, developed an acceptable bipolar lead.[13] William Chardack and Wilson Greatbatch adapted it for their version of a pacemaker system, abandoning work with their own troubled electrodes. Because of the time saved by that decision, they secured primacy in implanting a long-term, self-contained system.

William Chardack and Wilson Greatbatch
Buffalo, New York, USA

Wilson Greatbatch was an extraordinary engineer with determination that matched that of Zoll and Belgard in the fully-contained, self-sufficient pacemaker race. Greatbatch was so determined that he worked in isolation within a wood-heated barn on his property. He set aside a $2,000 research and development fund and gave his wife enough money to run the household. Within two years, Greatbatch produced 50 hand-made pacemakers. Through the efforts of William Chardack, chief of thoracic surgery at the Veteran Affairs Hospital in Buffalo, New York, 40 were placed in animals and 10 in patients. After doing the math, Greatbatch concluded that each of his $40 implantable pacemakers was an all-time bargain in the history of medical electronics.[14] Following successful testing of their pacemakers in animals, Chardack and Greatbatch reported their results at surgical society meetings and then published their paced animal experience. To prove their claim of being the first to implant a fully contained, self-sustaining pacemaker in a human ahead of close competitors Zoll and Kantrowitz, they added an unusual post script to their article about animal pacing experiments. The postscript cited successful pacemaker implantation in three patients.[15] The report caught the attention of the medical community. The first patient, reported as F.H., was Frank Henefelt,[16,17] a 75-year-old, football-helmeted former employee of a rubber company who experienced four blackouts the previous year – one caused a skull fracture. In the first stage of his pacemaker operation, on April 18, 1960, Chardack implanted the wire electrodes developed by Hunter and Roth in Minneapolis; the tips of the electrodes were secured to the surface of the heart muscle and their ends drawn through the anterior abdominal wall. Chardack temporarily attached them to an external pacer. After an observation period of about 50 days that established the Hunter-Roth electrode's stability, Chardack performed the second stage of the operation. On June 6, 1960, he shortened the external portions of the electrodes and attached a self-contained pacemaker made by Greatbatch. The joined components of the completed system were then implanted deep within the undersurface of the abdominal skin.

William Glenn and Alexander Mauro
New Haven, Connecticut, USA

While laying plans for a long-term fully-contained pacemaker in 1955, Paul Zoll and Alan Belgard experimented with radiofrequency technology that was less cumbersome, "fairly reliable" and surgically less demanding. The method was developed by physiologist Alexander Mauro at Yale University and adapted to patients at Grace New Haven Community Hospital in 1959 by surgeon William Glenn.

Glenn's first recipient, identified as W.T. in the medical literature, was

William Tobbler,[18] a 72-year-old retired executive who suffered for three years with symptomatic complete heart block that rate accelerant medication failed to stabilize. He was sent home attached to a line-operated external pacemaker, making Mr. Tobbler a rare example of a patient with a line-operated transthoracic external pacer used in a home setting.[19] But Tobbler could not tolerate the pain associated with closed-chest pacing, so he permitted its use only at low voltages that were usually ineffective.[20] William Glenn needed another approach for his patient.

A possible option was to attach a wire directly to the heart and run the wire outside the body to an external pacer. For concerns similar to those expressed by Äke Senning in Sweden, William Glenn refused to pace the heart with wires that penetrated through skin because infection is a predictable, inevitable outcome. The perpetual battle between "bugs" and man is a standoff only if the skin shield remains intact. Any scratch that breaches that barrier invites access to invaders that can rot flesh. An externalized pacer wire goes even deeper, providing a portal of entry to a being's innermost core. Glenn recognized that in the event of infection, antibiotic treatment to eliminate all bacteria imbedded in the internal plastic or metallic components of a pacing system would be futile, and that all "hardware" would have to be removed.

Glenn subsequently asked Alexander Mauro about his ideas for a pacer system that would not compromise the integrity of the skin shield. Based on his work as a physiologist, Mauro recommended that Glenn try radiofrequency pacing of the heart. Mauro had already used a radiofrequency device to broadcast through the skull to the brain[21] and it is likely that he was familiar with other applications of the method.[22] A radiofrequency transmitter can communicate with a receiver through one or two centimeters of skin. The Mauro-Glenn radiofrequency pacer systems consisted of two electrodes attached to the outer surface of the heart that terminated at a small radio receiver with an antenna implanted under the skin of the anterior chest. Mauro's early antennae were fashioned from electroencephalogram recording wires manufactured by the Grass Company. Outside of the body, a line-operated external radiofrequency transmitter sent a continuous stream of pulsed signals through a coil that adhered to the surface of the chest overlying the receiver's antenna. Each signal directed at the receiver triggered an electrical impulse that was passed on to stimulate the heart via its direct connection by cardiac wires. Pacing failed if the coil strayed too far from the site of the implanted antenna. Subsequent models of the transmitter were powered by batteries, doing away with the electrical cord plugged into a wall socket.

The commitment from Glenn's team to explore uncharted territory boosted Tobbler's hopes while he lay in hospital experiencing Stokes-Adams seizures and fearing a need of the dreaded transthoracic pacer at his bedside.[23] Glenn and his desperate patient knew that death might follow the last or the next heartbeat. Glenn also recognized that there wasn't time to pretest Mauro's pacemaker in animals, so he rushed ahead with the implant without the customary trials.[24] The drama intensified on January 29, 1959, when Tobbler had to be revived from a cardiac arrest in the operating room during the procedure. The radiofrequency system worked well in the immediate and early post-operative periods. Although the vacuum-tube transmitter was powered by line voltage, a backup system powered by a storage battery kept the pacemaker operational during a New Haven power outage on the third recuperative day.[25,26] When a wire fracture disabled the system on the 20th day, Tobbler remained stable, refused another operation and was discharged to his home on the 30th day. But he lacked Arne Larsson's good luck. A fatal attack soon extinguished William Tobbler's life. He was among the courageous pioneer patients in desperate circumstances who volunteer for untried procedures. They are often under-appreciated. Praise is usually directed elsewhere.

William Glenn and Alexander Mauro put disappointment behind them and moved forward. As a colleague of Glenn later described it, "To persist you have to have enormous personal courage … both the patient and the surgeon was being courageous as they underwent this procedure together … These patients had no alternative. Bill Glenn would sit for hours preoperatively and postoperatively to describe the procedure of what we were going to do … He was a remarkable man."[27] Glenn perfected his surgical technique and Mauro miniaturized the radiofrequency transmitter with transistors and batteries. They published an article describing a series of eight patients in 1962[28] and another with 17 patients in 1964.[29] The first eight implants had six electrode failures. Because Glenn was further along the learning curve of experience during the second series, there was a dramatic improvement with only two electrode failures. For a while, Glenn's electrodes were made of donated Elgiloy, a patented alloy used for main springs in Elgin watches.[30] The electrode failures experienced by Glenn remain a perpetual problem. Today's device companies continue to search for their Holy Grail – the elusive ideal electrode.

Paul Zoll and Alan Belgard
Experiments with radiofrequency pacing and the clinical implantation of long-term, self-contained "permanent" pacemakers
Boston, Massachusetts, USA

For approximately two years between 1958 and 1960, Paul Zoll tested the radiofrequency concept in animals[31-35] while simultaneously striving to be the first to develop and implant a long-term, fully self-contained pacer system in a human. The radiofrequency system uniformly failed because the voltage energy requirements to stimulate the heart gradually increased above the capacity that the pacemaker could deliver. Although a technical advance, clearly the radiofrequency pacer was flawed. For a while its many faults were overlooked because there were no reliable alternatives. Before radiofrequency stimulation was abandoned, it was applied to the phrenic nerve for diaphragmatic paralysis and to implantable transvenous endocardial pacing systems for heart block in children.[36] Zoll never tried it in a patient because he wasn't able to stabilize the energy requirements of the leads. He cautioned others, "…devices that depend on externally applied components are fundamentally too unsafe to be used in patients who have so treacherous an illness as Stokes-Adams disease." Zoll ended with an example of his dry wit, "We have to have something that nobody, particularly doctors can fool with."[37]

At long last, Paul Zoll succeeded in suppressing the rise in pacing thresholds after reading an article in a Corning publication that implicated sterile particles on the epicardial lead that could incite a scar at the interface between the heart muscle and the pacemaker lead. Such barrier scars gradually reduce myocardial responses to electrical stimulation as higher and higher pacemaker voltage output is needed to penetrate through the impediment. Armed with that new knowledge, Zoll and thoracic surgeon Howard Frank devised a lengthy operating-room ritual that stabilized pacing thresholds. The centerpiece was to boil the leads with their attached curved needles for 15 minutes in a large beaker

of water that contained
Ivory Flakes detergent.
After boiling, the leads
were thoroughly rinsed
with distilled water. The
process might have been
more magical than scien-
tific – but it worked.[38,39]
Paul and his reliable
surgeon, Howard Frank,
pressed on even though
they knew that their
effort would be "without
the reward of priority."[40]
The Beth Israel team's
initial epicardial lead
implant was three
months after that of

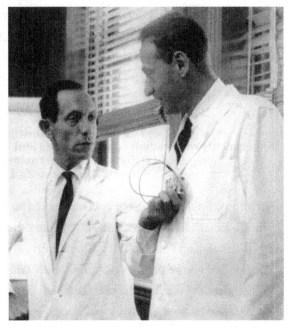

Paul Zoll holding a prototype Electrodyne self-contained
implantable pacemaker at the chest–level of implanting surgeon,
Howard Frank. Circa 1960. Courtesy of the Ruth and David Freiman
Archives at Beth Israel Deaconess Medical Center. With permission.

Chardack and Greatbatch's on Frank Henefelt, who later had a self-contained
pacer implanted. Frank and Zoll completed stage two (pacer implantation) on
their index patient almost five months after Henefelt's second stage procedure.
Zoll and Frank's first long-term, implantable pacer patient was a journeyman
physician who traveled from Canada to Boston seeking salvation from
disabling, unpredictable fainting spells. Named Michael Seiffer, he was a
62-year-old, Polish-born British subject who on April 13, 1959, collapsed on a
bus in England and self-diagnosed a Stokes-Adams attack.[41] While working in
Le Pas, Manitoba, a medically remote patch on the Canadian map, intermittent
recurrences resulted in his admission to the local hospital that served Eskimos
and indigenous Indians. Coincidentally, an airplane carrying a group of
American medical doctors to a convention in western Canada encountered
motor trouble, forcing an unscheduled landing at the La Pas airstrip. Faced with
a long delay, the group trekked off to the local hospital to pass the time. By
serendipity, the doctors came upon patient Michael Seiffer and his sad history
of persistent unpredictable fainting spells, even while on appropriate

medication. Some among the visitors indicated that Paul Zoll might be ready to undertake a compassionate clinical effort for such a patient.[42] The president of the Manitoba Medical Society concurred that a new approach, like an implanted pacemaker, was appropriate. Seiffer stabilized long enough to travel to Boston.

After arrival, his condition reverted to five or six attacks each day. Dr. Seiffer, knowing that he had a lethal illness, was preparing to die while wanting to live. He persuaded an uncomfortable and reluctant Zoll to prematurely move forward with a pacer implantation. Paul recorded his reservations, writing that "Seiffer urged us to operate without delay because of his desperate state."[43] Paul Zoll's intuition was correct. On July 20, 1960, during preliminary skin scrubs and draping procedures, the doctor/patient had a cardiac arrest. Unperturbed, surgeon Howard Frank promptly opened the chest, massaged the stilled heart, secured the electrodes to the exposed muscle of the left ventricle and exteriorized the wires to an external pacemaker.[44,45] Seiffer was none the worse from the crisis. Leona Zarsky remembered the reanimated patient on a heart monitor watching a baseball game the next day. "His heart slowed, and then responded to the pacemaker. The patient recovered and went home tied to the pacemaker against any of his physicians' hopes,"[46] Dr. Zarsky later explained.

After an observation period confirming that the leads' pacing thresholds were satisfactory and stable, the exposed external heart wires were sterilized with solutions and attached to a prototype Electrodyne fully self-contained, long-term pacemaker. The system was implanted in Seiffer's upper abdomen just below the ribcage on October 28, 1960.[47] It was the world's second pacer implant of its kind. Was Paul Zoll disappointed for not being the first? If so, disappointment was mitigated by satisfaction for completing a 12-year mission to spare victims of Stokes-Adams disease from disability or death. However, the thrill of that victory was soon replaced by the agony of a setback. An edge of the prototype pacemaker, which was potted in a container originally intended to hold a package of cigarettes, eroded through the skin, causing an infection and the need to exteriorize (externalize) the pacemaker unit. In time a new pacemaker was re-implanted. During the years that followed, Dr. Seiffer intermittently returned from Canada to have his system revised. When dormant bacterial infection flared, the implanted Electrodyne pacer was removed and the heart wires attached to an external pacemaker supported in a pouch.

Despite such difficulties, Seiffer regarded Paul Zoll and Howard Frank as saviors. In one act of gratitude, the patient designated Howard Frank sole beneficiary on an accidental death and disability insurance policy when departing from Boston's Logan Airport en route to Canada. Dr. Seiffer lived by the advice he offered to fellow sufferers of medical illness. "Have faith in God who will never let you down and have faith in your doctor who will do his best to help you."[48]

Overall, Paul Zoll's first case was a sweet, turned bitter experience. The procedure was a short-term success, but failed its purpose as a long-term pacemaker that could afford Seiffer a carefree unrestricted lifestyle. His occasional externalized electrodes were a threatening portal for potential bacterial invasion.

Unfortunately, the shaky start of Paul Zoll's implantable pacemaker program did not end with Dr. Seiffer – although it was ironic that the next mishap involved the doctor rather than the patient. Zoll's second patient, known as F.B., had an 18-month history of Stokes-Adams attacks that necessitated hospital treatment in Altoona, Pennsylvania. Zoll's request to transfer F.B. to Boston was denied by the Altoona attending physician because unmonitored travel with a continuous intravenous infusion of isoproterenol intended to increase heart rate was simply too risky. Undeterred, Paul drove to Altoona in his old Ford, collected the patient while attached to his intravenous drip and headed back to Boston. En route they stopped for lunch at a roadside diner. The server took their order without noticing the intravenous bottle hanging on a coat hook beside their booth. Upon returning with the order, the waitress noticed the infusion bottle, became alarmed, and dropped her precariously balanced tray of food on Paul. Otherwise, the trip was without incident.[49] On August 09, 1960, while in the operating room being prepared for implantation of epicardial leads, F.B.'s heart fibrillated immediately after intubation. The cardiac arrest was once again masterfully managed by Howard Frank.[50] On November 7, 1960, Dr Frank implanted a long-term pacemaker. The remainder of the course was uneventful.

Adrian Kantrowitz
Maimonides Hospital
Brooklyn, New York, USA

Adrian Kantrowitz, Chief of Surgery at Maimonides Hospital in Brooklyn, New York, was the third pioneer to implant a self-contained permanent pacemaker. The device he used came from a collaborative effort involving the Maimonides Hospital Surgical Research Division and the Advanced Circuit Division of General Electric.[51] Kantrowitz became interested in building a pacemaker after reading about an electronic metronome in the journal Popular Science. The same 1958 article was the creative spark that prompted Earl Bakken to invent a battery operated external pacer for Walton Lillehei in Minnesota. Kantrowitz assembled some pacemakers from parts purchased at a cluster of stores on lower Manhattan's Canal Street. He then tested the devices in dogs before considering a clinical trial. His first patient to have a self contained pacemaker was Rose Cohen, a 46-year-old woman who suffered from multiple Stokes-Adams attacks. She too endured the additional indignity of wearing a football helmet for protection during fainting spells while awaiting a cure.[52] Adrian Kantrowitz and Rose Cohen are another example of a courageous doctor and a desperate patient favoring an untried or unconfirmed treatment. Just as Rune Elmqvist and Äke Senning had Arne Larsson, Seymour Furman and John Schwedel had Pinkus Shapiro, William Glenn and Alexander Mauro had William Tobbler, William Chardack and Wilson Greatbatch had Frank Henefelt, Paul Zoll and Howard Frank had Michael Seiffer, at Maimonides Hospital Adrian Kantrowitz had Rose Cohen.

Her first operation occurred on September 28, 1960. Dr Kantrowitz secured electrodes to her heart and brought the wires through her skin to an external pacemaker. It is unclear if Kantrowitz had any intention of performing a two-stage procedure that would require his later implanting an internal pacemaker. His handmade units were tested in dogs, but never used in man. Perhaps Kantrowitz considered them not ready for human use. After Rose Cohen's electrode wires fractured and she experienced several other system failures with the external configuration, Kantrowitz consulted with engineers from General Electric. The engineers judged Kantrowitz's pacemaker to be ultra primitive and set about improving it.[53] The result was a self-contained, long-term implantable pacemaker that could be rate altered with an external programming device. A Kantrowitz-General Electric prototype total system was implanted in Rose on March 22, 1961.[54] The schematic on the next page illustrates the different approaches of Chardack, Zoll and Kantrowitz.

Paul Zoll and Howard Frank
Rewiring the Heart

Paul Zoll and Howard Frank were an inseparable team. During open-chest pacer implant procedures, Paul stood at the shoulder of Howard monitoring and managing heart rhythm as he had during World War II when Dwight Harken removed shrapnel from within and about the hearts of wounded soldiers. Years later, Harken – who was usually quick to criticize fellow surgeons – gave Howard Frank his highest accolade, stating that "Paul Zoll worked with Howard Frank, a brilliant surgical colleague." [55]

Like each of the other pioneer implant pacemaker surgeons, Zoll and Frank first used an open-chest exposure to place the leads on the heart's surface. However, with the Zoll/Frank team and some others, that procedure was most often replaced by a transvenous closed-chest approach that did not require direct exposure of the heart. Those long-term, catheter-electrode-based pacemaker procedures were more demanding on Paul Zoll's skills than either shrapnel recovery or open-chest pacer implants had been. That's because during the early, most hazardous part of such procedures, Paul often chose to maintain the heart rate of many patients with dilute solutions of cardiac rate accelerants rather than a temporary transvenous pacer electrode. After a long-term, permanent transvenous electrode was secured to the inner surface of its targeted heart chamber by a third team member who was a specially trained invasive cardiologist, Paul thoroughly tested every pacer system while Howard Frank awaited approval to start the final stages of the operation. Howard Frank, the invasive cardiologist, and Paul's patients greatly appreciated his supportive role.

In 1977, Zoll reflected on the circumstances that slowed progress in producing a reliable, fully implanted self-contained pacemaker. The problems were common to all pacemaker pioneers. Zoll's published comments start and end with Michael Seiffer. "He told us he couldn't wait to perfect our

Early Model Fully Contained Pacemakers

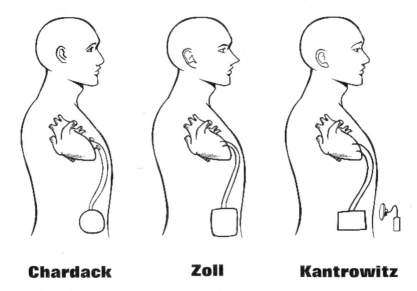

Chardack   Zoll   Kantrowitz

LEFT: Chardack/Greatbatch pacemaker with Hunter Roth leads
CENTER: Zoll/Belgard Electrodyne pacemaker with Electrodyne leads
RIGHT: Kantrowitz/General Electric pacemaker with GE leads and an external rate programmer

Original illustration above by Tim Prendergast, after Cammilli L, Pozzi R, De Saint Pierre G, Gallenga G, Menegazzo G. La stimolazione ellettrica del cuore nel trattamento del blocco atrio–ventricolare. L A Medicina Internazionale–N.7–1966.Page 56–57

instruments. He wanted a pacemaker to be put in at once … He lived for three years and died of complications of cardiac pacing that were so many in those days." In the article, Zoll elaborated on the past, engaged the present (1977) and expressed his hopes for the future. "Most of the complications have now been solved. They deal with displacement, fracture and infection of electrodes, with unreliable electronic components and circuitry, with inadequate energy sources, with leaky encapsulation. The major progress since those days has been the gradual, painfully slow, increasing reliability of the cardiac pacemaker-electrode system. We still have far to go in this primary task of making pacemakers entirely safe."[56]

In spite of many painful moments along his journey, Dr. Zoll fulfilled his vision of preventing sudden death associated with Stokes-Adams attacks. With the placement of Michael Seiffer's pacemaker in 1960, and those that followed, Paul completed a mission that started in 1948 when he lost an otherwise healthy

Stokes-Adams patient for lack of any known reliable therapy. Paul Zoll and his coworkers developed yet another method of reviving and maintaining a heart that stopped ticking by correcting Nature's imperfection with artificial wires and a power source.

FOURTEEN

THE FIRST CHILD WITH A TOTALLY IMPLANTED PACEMAKER

Paul Zoll was a close second to the Buffalo, New York, team of William Chardack and Wilson Greatbatch in a race to implant a self-contained pacemaker in an adult. In the more difficult task of placing a similar style pacemaker in a child, Zoll crossed the finish line just ahead of Chardack and Greatbatch.

High risk surgical correction of congenital heart disease in children became a reality in the late 1950s with the advent of hypothermia pioneered by Wilford Bigelow's Canadian team, heart bypass surgery, and a handful of courageous surgeons who were willing to help desperate kids. Many of the patients had a so called "hole in the heart" from a ventricular septal defect, which is an opening in the partition that separates the heart's main chambers (see figure on next page). These ventricular septal "hole in the heart" defects were among the earliest and most frequent to be operated upon in the mid 1950s. All the youngsters were extremely ill with prospects of dying in the near term. While closing the defect brought expectations of health and long life, too often during surgery the crucial electrical pathway between the small and the large heart chambers was temporarily injured or permanently severed because its location along a border of the hole made it vulnerable to transection by the surgeon's blade or strangulation by the surgeon's suture knot. In that circumstance, signals from the heart's natural pacemaker are ineffective in driving the main pumping chambers. An unreliable and slow subsidiary pacemaker takes over by default but it is much less effective than the primary pacemaker. The medical diagnosis is termed "heart block"–a condition that is difficult to treat in children because they are intolerant to rate-accelerating medications. Beginning in 1952, closed-chest Grass stimulator models similar to the one used by Paul Zoll were available,[1] and as early as 1954, advanced model Zoll-Electrodyne closed-chest pacemakers were in production. For six years, in the absence of an alternative, Zoll's painful method was essential to support the lives of children who suffered from post-operative heart block.

During the eight-year period that led up to Zoll's first-ever pacemaker implant in a child, several developments contributed to the breakthrough that brought hope and relief to the parents and to their children who had acquired accidental surgical heart block. It started with creative research at Harvard Medical School and its hospital affiliates. Judah Folkman, a brilliant student at Harvard Medical School from 1953 to 1957 with aspirations of becoming a surgeon, spent each summer vacation and all of his spare time in the laboratory of Robert Gross, the Chairman of Pediatric Surgery at Children's Hospital Boston.[2] Gross pioneered new approaches to correct many of nature's cardiac birth defects. While a student, Folkman addressed the problem of unintended

Ventricular Septal Defects

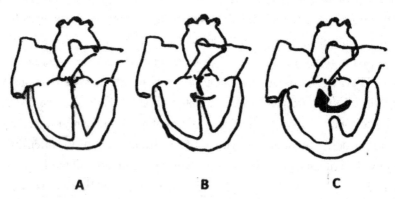

A   **B**   **C**

A: Normal heart. There is no communication between lower heart chambers. The separating septum is intact.
B: A small hole defect in the septum that permits low flow (arrow) from the heart's lower left chamber to the right chamber.
C: A large hole in the septum that allows high flow from the left to the right chamber. The strain on the heart enlarges the lower chambers and the pulmonary artery towards which the arrow is pointing. Larry Graves had a large defect.

complete heart block that often resulted from those corrective operations.[3] With the help of biomedical engineer Frederick Vanderschmidt at the Massachusetts Institute of Technology, Folkman developed an artificial pacemaker that permitted the main chambers of a dog's heart to respond to nature's true signal even in the presence of surgically created heart block. Folkman attached a pair of electrodes to the right-sided small chamber and another pair to the right-sided large heart chamber. The free end of each electrode pair was externalized and an amplifier-pacemaker was interposed in sequence between them. The ends of the atrial electrodes were connected to the amplifier for input, and the ventricular electrode pair was connected to the amplifier for output. Each amplified, small-chamber, atrial signal triggered a stimulus to excite the large chambers. The components of this *atrial signal amplifier that functioned as a ventricular pacemaker* were combined in a single unit that was strapped to the dog's outer body. It was the first *physiological* pacer system in the sense that the heart's small chamber drove its main chambers, as is Nature's way. Although the pacer was never used in a patient, it was a prototype for an advanced pacemaker design, making Folkman's animal experiments a proof of concept. In time, the "bugs" were eliminated, the concept was made patient-safe, miniaturized, commercialized and implanted in humans.[4] Also in time, Judah Folkman fulfilled his early aspirations when he succeeded Robert Gross as chair of pediatric surgery at Children's Hospital Boston. He arrived "at the center of leading-edge medicine." [5]

Another major contribution came from Walton Lillehei in Minnesota. Lillehei was dismayed by an unacceptably high rate of heart block that complicated his closures of ventricular septal defects. He was frustrated by the failure of rate accelerant medications to sustain improvement, the limitations of closed-chest pacing, and the near universal death rate in his patients with persistent heart block. Interdisciplinary cross fertilization of ideas catalyzed a solution in 1956. In that year, a Boston-trained professor of physiology named John A. Johnson attended a Lillehei case review of a post-surgery heart block death. Johnson had already spent a post-graduate year in Otto Kreyer's Harvard Medical School research laboratory. After hearing the account, Johnson asked Lillehei and his team to consider placing a detachable electrode on a main heart chamber at the conclusion of surgery. If needed, the heart would be stimulated through the electrode by an external pacemaker. Johnson had used this technique and a Grass stimulator in frog-heart experiments at the Harvard Medical School research laboratory.[6]

Two of Lillehei's junior associates, William Weirich and Vincent Gott, fast tracked the technique in their mentor's research laboratory. The procedure worked in animals and in Lillehei's post-operative heart block infants. As a result, his Minnesota group became the first in the world to attach an electrode to a human heart and drive it from an external stimulator. Judah Folkman of Harvard and Walton Lillehei published their findings on the same date in the same journal.[7,8] Lillehei's pacing method, introduced in 1958, became standard temporary treatment for surgically induced heart block. It almost totally replaced Paul Zoll's closed-chest pacing technique – an approach that had been in place since 1952.

Buffalo, New York, and Boston versions of a long-term implantable pacemaker were good solutions for permanent heart block. Their success led to Zoll's first implant in a child near the end of 1960.

Larry Wayne Graves, an eight-year-old from far away Fairmont, West Virginia, was the fourth patient in Paul Zoll's implanted pacemaker series.[9] Larry was a sickly child who failed to thrive since his birth on May 27, 1952. He often wished that he could be like his robust twin brother, Barry Layne Graves. Their father and the breadwinner of the family, Thomas, worked for Westinghouse. He and his wife, Barbara Ann, had four children, two foster children, a modest house with a mortgage and a car. They were salt of the earth proud folks who were able to meet their financial obligations if the family remained in good health.[10] But Larry's lack of growth and strength became a high level concern. The cause of the condition was unclear until the wise family doctor, suspecting congenital heart disease, suggested that Larry be examined at Children's Hospital Boston, where pioneering corrective surgery was being performed by Robert Gross and members of his department. Little Larry first became a patient there at age 22 months.[11] His struggle with a weak heart involved a devoted family, the support of local and distant communities, courageous collaborative doctors and a hospital with a heart that treated the hearts of children.

Larry was just approaching his second year of life when he was admitted to Children's Hospital Boston and diagnosed with a ventricular septal defect. Doctors advised his parents to defer surgery as long as possible because operations on older children were known to have better outcomes and higher survival rates. At age eight, weighing only 40 pounds, Larry's fragile condition became critical. His parents, already suffering financially under the weight of his medical expenses, were determined to save their child, literally "at all cost." They returned to Boston with Larry. The Graves' three other children and two foster children remained in West Virginia in the care of a relative.[12] On October 14, 1960, Dr. Samuel Schuster and a team of surgeons at Children's Hospital closed the septal defect. By chance, it was accompanied by the dreaded complication – heart block. Cardiac rate control was maintained by the Lillehei method powered by an Electrodyne automatic pacemaker system that had its ancestral incandescence in Otto Kreyer's Harvard Medical School laboratory bordering Children's Hospital, and from Paul Zoll's pacemaker works in a Beth Israel Hospital laboratory across the street. Robert Gross, the leader of pediatric surgery with comprehensive knowledge of complex and current pacing practices, knew that restoration of Larry's heart conduction was possible if "time would only heal." Thomas and Barbara Ann waited, hoped and prayed while lodged in facilities paid for by workers of the local Westinghouse union affiliate, whose members also had donated blood.[13] Heart block persisted, was unremitting and was dangerous. On November 10, 1960, Howard Frank (the surgical partner of Paul Zoll during every pacemaker implantation) and Samuel Schuster (a Children's Hospital staff surgeon) led a team that placed a self-contained Electrodyne pacing system in a single-stage procedure at Children's. The large pacemaker was positioned in the left flank near the kidney. Because Larry Graves' operation was completed in one-stage, his totally internalized "permanent" pacemaker was functioning flawlessly when he left the operating room.

Larry's procedure was completed the same month as Chardack and Greatbatch's 13th case in Buffalo, when a seven-year old had lead placement only, which is the first step of a two-stage procedure.[14] The second stage, needed to complete the system, required the placement of a pacemaker after determining that the leads were stable – a determination that varies in time from weeks to months. The delay gave Larry Graves the gravitas of being the first child in the world to receive a long-term pacemaker. It also gave Paul Zoll primacy in another first-in-the-world achievement, although the accomplishment was one that he never publicized.

Happily for publicity-shunning Paul Zoll, media coverage that followed the barrier-breaking surgery shed some limelight on Howard Frank (1914-2004). Howard was an eclectic academic surgeon with wide-ranging interests, such as the importance of Vitamin K in blood coagulation,[15] more than a decade-long investigation of traumatic and surgical shock,[16,17] peritoneal irrigation in renal failure,[18] guide-wire location of non-palpable breast tumors,[19] thoracic and heart surgery, and innovative techniques in pacemaker implantation, including management of a broad spectrum of post operative complications that plagued surgeons and their patients.[20,21] He is best remembered as a pioneer pacemaker surgeon. After Children's Hospital issued a news release two weeks following the milestone operation, the media spread the word and reported on Larry's progress. Articles appeared in the November 28, 1960, edition of Newsweek,[22] and in the March 4, 1961, edition of the Saturday Evening Post. Larry's story and his cheerful appearance captivated the nation. A local reporter misrepresented the facts by mentioning Howard Frank as the sole surgeon. The error was perpetuated by others. In a letter to co-implant surgeon Sam Schuster, Howard expressed his anger and dismay, "Horrors! You would think I did the damned operation."[23] A copy went to the directorship of Children's. A magnanimous reply followed to the effect that any improvement in Larry's health, or any extension of his life, would be due entirely to Howard's effort.[24]

Larry was still recovering at Children's Hospital during Thanksgiving, 1960. Gifts flowed his way. He shared them with his siblings. After discharge Larry revisited Boston to correct pacemaker complications or for routine visits. The family received financial assistance from Westinghouse workers. The news media followed Larry's progress and setbacks. There were exaggerated reports of a deep-in-debt family becoming destitute, the need to sell the furniture, loss of the car and possibly the house.[25] In West Virginia, the Fairmont Woman's Club established a fund. With local industry in decline, neighbors donated what little they could. Boston papers listed the Fairmont donation address. At the

outset, inmates at the Massachusetts State
Prison in Walpole raised money and presented
gifts to Larry, explaining, "We want to help in
our own small way. ...we are all in your
corner pulling for you."[26] The hospital
medical bill was defrayed by private donations
and the balance forgiven.[27] The family moved
to an affordable town near Boston to be close
to the primary source of Larry's care. Boston
hospitals in general and Children's Hospital in
particular are known as places where
materialism yields to human compassion. A
close affiliate of Children's, the House of the
Good Samaritan (1924-1973) was an 80-bed
hospital with a mission to treat ill children.
It always rendered care without charge.[28]

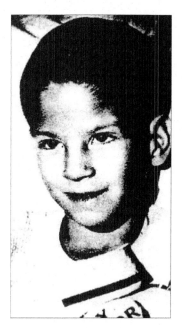

Larry Graves while recovering in
Children's Hospital after long-term
pacemaker placement. From the
article *Hearten Heart Boy* that
appeared in the Boston Daily
Record, December 19, 1960.
Used with permission of the
Boston Herald.

When Larry's worst moments were
behind him, Thomas reflected "We have
faith... Larry has been spared for a reason."[29]

As a sad post script, Larry Graves died of
heart failure on June 17, 1989, at the age of 37. Prior to corrective surgery, he
had envied twin brother Barry's vigor and his ability to participate in athletics.
But Barry died even earlier, in a January 1981 auto accident at the age of 29.

Placing pacemakers in children was, and continues to be, a formidable
challenge. In 1964, a worldwide review reported only 17 children with implanted
pacemakers in contrast to 1,499 adults.[30] The first recipient, Larry Graves, was
near death at the age of eight, when his life was spared by Robert Gross' surgical
division at Children's Hospital and Paul Zoll's pacemaker team at Beth Israel
Hospital. Although Paul did not wish to be remembered for his fully implantable
pacemaker, he derived great satisfaction in witnessing its life-normalizing and
life-sparing properties.

FIFTEEN

CARDIOVERSION DISPLACES COUNTERSHOCK

In the early 1960s, the medical landscape became a battleground between direct current (DC) and alternating current (AC) shock for resetting cardiac arrhythmias. Bernard Lown led the invading forces of DC defibrillation, while Paul Zoll valiantly defended his territory, favoring the AC method of countershock that he had pioneered with his first successful defibrillation in 1955 (see figure, Chapter 10, page 63). Even when his followers deserted en mass, Zoll refused to surrender and stuck to his guns for years. It wasn't until the late 1970s that he finally acknowledged that DC shock was the only way to power initiatives for future electrocardiac therapy. In the intervening years, the clinical term *countershock*, which Zoll had introduced to describe his use of AC to reset heart rhythm, was displaced by the word *cardioversion*, the term Lown introduced to describe resetting by DC.[1]

The controversy between Zoll and Lown echoed an earlier mammoth battle, also laced with rancor, which raged during the late 1800s to determine if alternating current or direct current would be distributed across America. In that case George Westinghouse's AC prevailed over Thomas Edison's DC to become the national standard.[2] The primary advantage of AC was that it could be more efficiently transmitted over long distances.

Some 75 years later, in the arguments between AC defibrillation and DC defibrillation, the DC approach won out because it enabled synchronized defibrillation shocks to occur during the safest part of the heart's electrical cycle. Alternating current defibrillation could not be timed with such accuracy.

Another advantage was that battery power commonly provided a DC source for fully implantable defibrillators.

However, there is no question that alternating current could succeed at doing the job during closed-chest or open-chest applications. There are even rare anecdotal reports of municipal AC electrification successfully terminating ventricular fibrillation in some unconventional, improbable, and desperate instances. At the time when Claude Beck first performed life saving open-chest defibrillation of a human in 1947, apparently very few operating rooms were equipped with defibrillators. Therefore, seven months after Beck's initial success, no such device was on hand when a patient undergoing an open-chest lung operation in Trenton, New Jersey, went into ventricular fibrillation. Lacking a defibrillator, the surgeon detached an electrical cord from the base of a lamp, stripped the outer covering and separated the two strands that lay within. He applied the open end of each wire at a distance from the other on the exposed heart. The surgeon then momentarily inserted the plug into a wall outlet. Against all odds, the AC shock restored normal rhythm.[3]

In another instance, Dr. Philip Gold recalled being an unexpected savior while on night duty at a satellite hospital of McGill University, Montreal, Canada, during medical residency training in 1963. A nurse called Gold to "come and pronounce a patient dead." He found a middle-aged man without pulse, with gasping respirations and with dilating pupils. Gold started vigorous external cardiac massage and rescue mouth-to-mouth ventilation, procedures he had recently learned from a training film produced at John Hopkins University.[4] Because the hospital did not own a defibrillator, Gold instructed the nurse to bring an electrocardiograph (ECG) machine and an electric cord severed from the base of a lamp. The ECG revealed ventricular fibrillation. Gold then prepared the cord in the same manner as the surgeon in Trenton, New Jersey, had done, except that Gold fashioned aluminum foil into paddle shapes and attached them to the bare ends of the electric cord's separated, negative and positive strands. The patient was intubated and the foil paddles positioned on his bare chest. Gold then had the plug inserted into an AC wall receptacle for approximately two seconds. Fibrillation persisted. He repositioned the paddles and repeated the procedure, this time with success. Fibrillation was replaced with unstable heart block that required external pacing.[5,6] Rib fractures were stabilized in the operating room by Harvey Sigman, the chief surgical resident, who decided to implant a long-term pacer the next day. The patient objected, became obstinate and refused to sign the consent. He acquiesced after Sigman, on instructions from his senior attending surgeon, threatened to turn off the life-sustaining external temporary pacemaker.[7]

While those tales concern interesting special cases, as a rule the worldwide experience after Paul Zoll's 1955 discovery of closed-chest AC countershock established AC defibrillation as a standard practice that restored life to multitudes of people who otherwise were destined to die. Zoll prevailed over adversaries schooled in open-chest resuscitation and doubters who branded an electrical close-chest cardiac revival impossible.

Ironically, after the appearance of the DC defibrillator in 1962, Zoll's customary role was reversed. He no longer strove to expand the borders of his well-deserved territorial conquests by convincing still skeptical minds that electrical resuscitation works. Now, he found himself defending what had become a gold-standard practice over the course of the prior six years.

The Assault

Closed-chest DC defibrillation had been historically successful in animals. Barouh Berkovits, a brilliant biomedical engineer, made the prodigious leap to building a DC defibrillator for clinical use. While Berkovits was the force behind the DC defibrillator in the western world, being the innovator, the inventor and modifier of the DC defibrillator that resets life-threatening and hazardous arrhythmias, he remained a modest hero. Born in Czechoslovakia in 1926, Berkovits stayed in that country until he received an engineering degree from Prague University in 1949. He then emigrated to Israel, where he held positions at the Hebrew University Physics Department and Hadassah Medical School. While in Israel, he assimilated all available information from academic scientific publications on electrocardiac therapy, harboring hopes to develop a better delivery system.[8,9] Berkovits concluded that a direct-current approach would be superior to the AC method then in use.

His next destination was the U.S.A., where he served as a senior engineer at Brooklyn Polytechnic Institute, followed by an appointment as Director of

Research at the Medical Division of the American Optical Company in Buffalo, New York. There he persuaded superiors that the theoretical superiority of a direct current defibrillator could lead the company to dominate the commercial market.

A casual conversation set the stage for animal and clinical trials. It occurred when Bernard Lown at the Harvard School of Public Health requested advice from American Optical in determining oxygen levels for a complex experiment. Berkovits met Lown. When asked, "What new things are you working on," Berkovits responded that he had invented a DC defibrillator. In a series of four letters that followed, between February 8 and May 5, 1961, Bernard Lown and his associate Sidney Alexander in essence related their views and experience with defibrillation, including dramatic success with AC elective countershock, poor knowledge of electronics and finally a formal request that Berkovits permit them to test his new DC defibrillator for efficacy in animals and for possible clinical application.[10,11] Barouh agreed and delivered his device.

Lown's comparative tests between DC and AC electroshock in animals demonstrated superiority of the Berkovits machine in terminating ventricular fibrillation, minimizing post-shock arrhythmias, and producing less measurable damage to the heart, including short-term complications and death. Barouh enhanced the efficacy of his defibrillator by having Lown experiment with three machines, each with a predetermined, fixed unique pulse wave and duration of delivery. Berkovits' so-called *underdamped* wave form was superior to the others, and a shorter delivery time was superior to those that were longer.[12]

Berkovits was familiar with the work of Wiggers and Wégria, who had mapped the electrical phases of the cardiac cycle and identified a period of vulnerability during which an applied stimulus could result in deadly fibrillation.[13] Carl Wiggers was the eminent cardiac physiologist at Western Reserve University, Cleveland, Ohio, who had been an early proponent of open-chest defibrillation in the 1940s. René Wégria was a collaborating scientist and close colleague of Wiggers. Their observation was later extended to native premature beats that strike during the vulnerable period of a preceding beat – concluding that whether natural or induced, a poorly timed impulse was potentially dangerous. The idea to time the defibrillator's discharge with the safest component of a heart beat's electrical phase appears to have come from

Berkovits. While he and Lown discussed avoiding the vulnerable period, to the best of Berkovits' recollection it was he (not Lown) who suggested that the defibrillator discharge be synchronized to the cardiac cycle.[14] Even if Lown did, or did not, initiate the idea, there is no doubt that he was a vehement proponent of synchronization. He was unmoved by Sidney Alexander's argument that a second shock would succeed in the event that a poorly timed initial shock induced an arrhythmia.[15] Alexander's solution echoed that of Paul Zoll.

While Berkovits enhanced defibrillator safety by introducing a timing circuit that allowed the operator to select the precise instant of electroshock to avoid the vulnerable period, Bernard Lown and his associates labored to create and implement experimental protocols to establish the safety and superiority of DC over AC. In reviewing his involvement with Lown and the DC defibrillator, Berkovits said, "I made it and he used it; " and "I invented it and he introduced it into clinical practice."[16] The patent for the synchronized defibrillator was filed on July 17, 1962, in Barouh Berkovits' name.

Lown's first clinical attempt with DC synchronized countershock occurred at a small hospital on the outskirts of Boston. The custom at the time was to perform the procedure with the patient under anesthesia in the operating room. Alcohol soaked sponges were erroneously placed under the paddles to serve as conductors. They exploded and burned when the synchronized defibrillator discharged.[17] It is said that we learn more from failure than from success. The mistake did not recur. Eight months later, Bernard Lown presented his findings at the 1962, 54th American Society of Clinical Investigation meeting in Atlantic City, New Jersey.[18] His conclusions, drawn from both the animal experiments and the clinical results of six patients, indicated that the DC method was superior and that AC was unsafe for use in humans.

Paul Zoll, seated in the audience, was unconvinced that DC shock was superior to AC. He perceived no advantage in an unconscious patient nearing death from ventricular fibrillation. In fact, he had been joined in that view by some investigators who found AC better than DC before optimal wave forms had been developed by Berkovits. In addition, Zoll believed that avoiding the vulnerable period was a non-issue. He argued that a stronger second countershock would correct a hazardous arrhythmia provoked by a previous attempt. After Lown's presentation in Atlantic City, Paul rose from his aisle chair, walked several feet to a microphone and questioned the validity of Lown's data and conclusions. A violent argument ensued. The content was either not recorded or has been sealed. Shocked witnesses cannot recall the specifics, only that neither party distinguished himself. According to one description, "Lown tried to outdo Zoll in being vituperative... It was clear that there was rancor on both sides."[19] A physician in training at the time recalled being told that Lown made Zoll look terrible.[20] According to an attendee seated near Paul Zoll, the verbal skirmish ended when someone in earshot of Zoll exclaimed in Yiddish, "Paul, sit down!"[21] A member of the Tulane contingent within arm's length of Paul told him, "Don't be upset with Bernard Lown, all he is doing is standing on your shoulders and looking a little farther, but the basic work is yours."[22] The incident was likely among the most memorable events of the scientific session. It continued to reverberate even after the meeting. Paul Axelrod, a future colleague of both Paul Zoll and Bernard Lown, recalled mention of the episode at the Ohio State University, Cardiology Division summary session of important presentations from Atlantic City.[23]

This was not the first time that Paul Zoll stepped out of character by violently disagreeing with an opposing point of view. He did so during a 1958 Rockefeller Conference when he "disagreed very violently" with any consideration of physiological pacing, which duplicates nature's sequence of heart chamber contraction by recruiting both small and large chambers, rather than the large ventricular chambers alone. The chairman soon thereafter called for a recess. When the session resumed, he reminded all participants that "violent" disagreements such as Zoll's were allowed as long as "mutual respect" was maintained. Nonetheless, Zoll's opponent retaliated by accusing Paul of "insulting mother nature."[24] When reflecting on the incident 15 years later, in 1973, Zoll recalled that he "objected in vain" because there was no way to apply the newly proposed complex technology without an effective pacing lead. That is why he favored sole, large chamber pacing.[25]

Paul Zoll and Bernard Lown were faculty at separate Harvard Medical School teaching hospitals. Their feud was perceived as an anomaly by most, but not all. Public disputes between physicians were not unheard of. Charles Bailey of Philadelphia and Harvard's Dwight Harken had public quarrels about technique and primacy in performing mitral valve surgery. Referring to Harken, Bailey said, "We had some differences of opinion. Besides that, Boston doctors fight at their medical meetings... He spoke after me and harshly criticized what I had done. I was shocked... "[26]

Meanwhile, advocates and evidence favoring DC resetting of arrhythmia continued to build. At the same 54th scientific session at which Zoll and Lown argued, Dwight Harken's group presented results comparing AC and DC defibrillation in closed-chest hypothermic dogs, along with three hypothermic open-chest operative patients. Direct current terminated ventricular fibrillation 98 percent of the time in animals compared to only 18 percent for AC. In all of the clinical cases, DC was an outstanding success. The premier success occurred in the first clinical case in which DC was tried. The patient, while still on the operating table, had failed to convert from ventricular fibrillation after 10 successive AC countershocks. Then, the first time Berkovits' DC defibrillator was used on the patient, ventricular fibrillation was terminated with a single shock.[27] That courageous effort was directed by Dwight Harken during desperate circumstances. In a familiar scenario, the DC defibrillator that finally proved successful was brought from Harken's distant research laboratory. The incident understandably shook his faith in AC defibrillation. After his stirring testimonial for DC defibrillation, Harken concluded his conference presentation in 1962 with a comment to the effect that, henceforth, AC defibrillators would be banished from his operating room. That ripple of discontent became a tsunami. Alternating current defibrillators were abandoned en mass. Most ended up in the junk heap. Others found homes in museums.

The Resistance

Paul Zoll continued to use AC defibrillation countershock because it worked well in his hands. In a 1964 letter to the editor of the Journal of the American Medical Association, Zoll defended AC life-sparing defibrillation and elective countershock for the lesser arrhythmias. His concise message was that AC and DC defibrillation were equivalent. Zoll argued that alternating current was completely safe and effective when properly applied. He wrote that failure or provocation of serious arrhythmias was rare with either AC or DC. Finally, Zoll insisted that the distinction between AC and DC was unimportant in clinical practice.[28] Even as the forces of general opinion overruled him, Zoll did not abandon AC. In 1967, five years after the introduction of DC cardioversion, he reported that 60-cycle unsynchronized AC of 0.15 second duration and a range of 150-750 volts remained his method of choice. In the same report, Zoll referred to failures of synchronized DC and believed that both types succeeded when used properly. He noted that he encountered only five instances of AC-induced ventricular fibrillation in more than 300 countershocks. Each instance was promptly terminated by another larger shock.[29] Paul Zoll stayed the course for years longer and in 1973 he suggested that the term *countershock* be preserved in preference to *defibrillation* because of the former's historic context. Zoll contended that other labels emanating from contemporary research laboratories should be avoided.[30] During his keynote Karel Frederik Wenckebach Memorial Lecture the same year, Zoll told the audience that he and some others disagreed with the current convention of calling countershock *synchronized cardioversion.*[31]

Throughout that period, Bernard Lown mounted a powerful ethical critique of Zoll's position on the grounds that, even if induced ventricular fibrillation could be reversed with a second shock, physicians treating a benign disorder should not endanger a patient in any way, including raising the risk of inducing ventricular fibrillation. Lown preached that synchronized DC cardioversion should always be used.[32]

Lown and Zoll had different temperaments that influenced their professional approaches. General impressions of trainees and physicians who worked with Lown and Zoll acknowledged those differences. They were summed up well by Paul Axelrod. He described Bernard Lown as highly organized, creative, and a master of language who obtained continuous funding that supported many trainees. Axelrod characterized Paul Zoll as very shy, with a familiarity of electronics that gave him insight and enabled direct involvement in developing his ideas. Zoll worked with limited funds and was more or less a loner.[33]

Yet Zoll also demonstrated a capacity to inspire people and help his trainees launch impressive careers. During one period of extraordinary productivity in the early 1950s, Paul Zoll had two post-graduate physician cardiology trainees and a research medical student. The physicians were Milton Paul and William Gibson. The medical student was Paul Minton, who later became an intern at Beth Israel Hospital. Milton Paul and William Gibson were co-authors with Zoll on major publications, which is the currency of academia. Milton Paul went on to a highly distinguished career as the Director of Pediatric Cardiology at Children's Hospital in Chicago. Before leaving Boston in 1958, he asked Zoll for an AC defibrillator to use in his pediatric cardiac catheter laboratory.[34] Milton later published a series describing children on whom his pre-owned AC machine was used to correct, by countershock, their "lesser," but compromising arrhythmias.[35] He might have been the first person to electively reset a child's serious arrhythmia. The report of the pediatric cases immediately followed Paul Zoll's description of elective AC termination of arrhythmias in adults.[36] Both reports appeared in the same issue of the same journal in 1962. In a later interview, Milton Paul described his time with Paul Zoll as "intoxicating." He recalled that solutions to problems were forthcoming all the time. Work in the laboratory was always moving forward and that everyone felt a sense of progress and accomplishment.[37]

William Gibson (1926-1988) is remembered as a hard worker with a wry sense of humor who enjoyed playing a tape recording of Tommy Dorsey when assigned to the research laboratory – the same Dorsey tape that medical student Paul Minton continuously played when he worked alone. William Gibson served in the military, practiced clinical cardiology in Detroit and was the first Afro-American to be board-certified in cardiology.

Paul Minton had a prior connection to Zoll before he studied with him. Minton's sister, a technician at Beth Israel Hospital, directed her entire family to Zoll for medical care. Minton started his career track as a biologist. But after earning a master's degree, he changed course and entered medical school. When Minton's mother learned from a casual remark by Zoll that he had a summer vacancy in his research laboratory, she recommended her son. Paul Minton was hired to work for Zoll between his first and second years of medical school. The experience was life-changing for the young student. Minton gained an internship at Beth Israel Hospital. With Zoll's encouragement and continued support, Paul Minton became an invasive cardiologist in the State of Maine.[38]

The Concession

While Paul Zoll believed that AC and DC were on a par, he initially overlooked the broader applications of DC. When it became clear that portable battery-powered defibrillators or combined defibrillator/pacemakers were needed at the points of care outside of hospitals, and that some clairvoyant scientists were developing internal defibrillators with powerful long-lasting lithium batteries, Paul's self-confessed stubbornness softened. When returning home from a Purdue Defibrillation Conference (circa 1978), he told his son, Ross, that DC would dominate the medical electronic industry.[39,40]

At that time, portable light-weight synchronized DC defibrillators had already been designed and refined in Belfast, Ireland, by John Anderson, biomedical engineer at the Royal Victoria Hospital. The early non-synchronized defibrillators, and later models, were applied clinically by Drs. Pantridge and Geddes from 1967 through 1970.[41,42] Technological advances continue to the present day. Automated external defibrillators (AED) represent the current state of the art. Although they are DC synchronized units, they are extensions of Paul Zoll's original vision.

Michel Mirowski, another visionary, believed in a fully implanted standby defibrillator that would be patient-safe, reliable and a savior to those at high risk of sudden arrhythmic death. In an instant, vulnerable candidates would receive an internal shock to terminate life threatening ventricular fibrillation or tachycardia. In 1970 Michel Mirowski and Morton Mower of the Sinai Hospital of Baltimore, Maryland, published results of a preliminary feasibility study in animals with a defibrillator outside the body that delivered a shock directly to the heart through one transvenous electrode within the heart and another electrode on the surface of the heart.[43] The next step, in 1971, was a similar mixed feasibility study with transvenous intravascular wire leads within the heart and an external defibrillator.[44] At the outset, Mirowski acknowledged that he was at the beginning of a project that needed to be refined over time. He had to work out generic engineering problems related to arrhythmia sensing, battery longevity and device miniaturization. He also had to define an appropriate class of patients who were at high predictable risk to suffer a life-threatening arrhythmia. Those problems, and others, had to be solved before moving on to a clinical trial of an implantable device. Progress was slow and deliberate. The first animal trial of the *implantable* defibrillator was in 1978[45] and the first report of three patients came in 1980.[46]

Mirowski's vision was in the historic tradition of implanted devices evolving from external ancestors, as they had with pacemakers, and also in the tradition of great ideas encountering resistance along the way. Long before the first animal implantation came to pass, Bernard Lown – by this time an authority on DC defibrillation – found Mirowski's concept in the cross hairs of his gun sight, pulled the trigger and fired a volley. Lown was skeptical of an internal defibrillator's safety and need. He enlisted the aid of Paul Axelrod, his cardiology colleague and biomedical engineer.[47] A report about their concerns, published in 1972, addressed specific technical and safety requirements of an implanted standby defibrillator plus the philosophical issues of societal cost, the ethics of placing a patient into ventricular fibrillation to test the device and the need for such an instrument. The publication concluded that the defibrillator was an imperfect gadget in search of a clearly defined application.[48]

Undeterred, Michel Mirowski, like Paul Zoll, was an unstoppable man on a mission. Constructive and destructive criticism drove him to work harder.[49] A supporter of Mirowski's effort, Zoll had not forgotten the harsh resistance he had overcome in his attempts to closed-chest pace or defibrillate the heart. Nor did he forget his long struggle to perfect the implantable pacemaker after the first primitive model. Zoll was pleased with the prospect of an internalized defibrillator.[50] Barouh Berkovits also supported Mirowski, "We spoke about it. I thought it was a good idea. It was needed."[51]

Overall, the period between 1960 and 1970 was Paul Zoll's decade to defend, refine, reinvent ideas and on occasion to recognize meritorious achievements of others that came "from elsewhere," such as DC defibrillators that morphed into AEDs and the implantable internal defibrillator.

SIXTEEN

REVISING OLD IDEAS, DISCOVERING NEW OPPORTUNITIES

A contrarian to Alexander Pope's advice "Be not first by whom the new are tried nor the last to lay the old aside,"[1] Paul Zoll cautiously introduced new methods into clinical practice and was likely the last to substitute a competing method "from elsewhere" for one of his successes. That reluctance was in consideration of the life and death consequences for patients, which caused Paul to place his primary trust in his own discoveries and observations – in the treatments that he knew would work from his own experience. Therefore he believed that his discoveries, even when superseded by new approaches, remained good, simple, and safe. That is why he considered them worthy of his continued praise and support. Paul's apparent stubbornness and healthy skepticism demanded long-term observation of benefit before his dissonance re-equilibrated.[2]

Throughout the course of his career, Paul resisted or resolved five new approaches proposed "from elsewhere," as summarized in the accompanying table on page 127. They primarily involved defibrillation, pacemaker design, pacemaker electrode placement, and emergency management of heart rate.

Defibrillation

Paul's confidence in his own experience and observations was evident during the spirited and contentious debate over direct current (DC) versus alternating current (AC), when Zoll, to his chagrin saw AC countershock displaced by DC cardioversion after his AC approach had been in the forefront during the decade

1952 to 1962. As noted in the preceding chapter, Zoll's position eventually softened with predictions by biomedical engineers that DC-generated wave forms would be used in all defibrillators, especially automated external and implanted internal devices, which would play an increasingly important role in preventing many sudden arrhythmic deaths.[3,4]

While Paul reluctantly accepted the predictions of the oracles and biomedical shamans, he was loath to abandon AC transthoracic countershock in his own practice, making him the last man standing to use an AC closed-chest defibrillator. Long before Paul Zoll's concession, Alan Belgard of Electrodyne – Zoll's collaborator in developing cardiac equipment – began accommodating his clients with DC defibrillators. He even stopped advertising AC defibrillators, but continued to deliver AC when ordered.[5]

Pacing On Demand

Implantable pacemakers developed in the late 1960s and 1970s featured multi-programmability that permitted two-chamber physiologic pacing (small chamber pacing followed by large chamber pacing), as well as the natural rhythm of small chamber activity followed by large chamber pacing. Among pacing options in the menu, there were "pacing on demand" modes that enabled pacing only when needed and theoretically prevented pacer stimuli from striking the cardiac vulnerable period.[6] Because Zoll had never encountered multiple response or ventricular fibrillation from a single stimulus strike during the vulnerable period, he believed that the issue was irrelevant. He also believed that the added pacer complexity introduced by the multi-programmability approach increased the possibility of device failure, which in turn compromised patient safety.[7,8]

For those reasons, Paul was adamant in promoting continuous, fixed, constant, non-programmable and factory set, single-rate large-chamber "permanent" pacing. Zoll was an occasional counterpoint panelist on cardiac management symposia such as Controversies In Cardiology. He argued that change is not always for the best. It is no surprise that Electrodyne manufactured all long term pacers in a dedicated, continuous, single-rate mode.

Zoll was not a solitary voice in the wilderness. Wilson Greatbatch also questioned the wisdom of abandoning fixed-rate continuous pacing. "It is

Changes Paul Zoll Resisted or Resolved

ISSUE	POPULAR VIEW	PAUL ZOLL'S VIEW
Emergency management of heart block, very slow or absent heart beat	• Rate-arousal medication • Transvenous temporary pacing	• Rate-arousal medication • Closed-chest pacing • Continuous low-dose intravenous cardiac accelerants
Ventricular fibrillation	DC shock	AC countershock
Lead placement with implanted pacemaker	Transvenous lead tip against inner wall of heart	• Open-chest procedure with leads placed in heart muscle from outer surface • Later changed to minimally invasive "fish hook" leads invented by Zoll/Frank
Complex implantable pacemakers	• On-demand pacing • Physiological pacing	Continuous single-rate pacing
Heart block, very slow or absent heart beat	• Rate-arousal medication • Transvenous temporary pacing • Re-evaluate	• Rate-arousal medication • New version closed-chest pacemaker • Re-evaluate

comforting to know that I am not completely alone in my opinion," wrote Greatbatch. He noted that he was in the good company of pioneers William Chardack, Paul Zoll and Adrian Kantrowitz.[9] It is noteworthy that neither Seymour Furman, a prime mover and advocate of transtelephonic pacemaker monitoring, nor Bernard Kosowski, another advocate, could recall a disaster during a telephonic pacer transmission, which often results in fixed-rate pacing with paced stimuli randomly striking the vulnerable period of native beats.[10]

Throughout the controversy, Paul invoked his experience, good results and the few exceptions that required him to modify old ideas. He presented his case succinctly, clearly and forcefully, but not persuasively enough to sweep back a rising tide of evidence with his broom. Over his objection, physiological pacing modes were among the most popular choices selected from each new generation of pacemaker's expansive multi-programmable menu. Demand pacing was a near universal choice, which even Paul eventually accepted in his practice. His one consolation was an option in the menu for continuous, fixed-rate pacing.

Pacer Electrode Placement

It is likely that long-term implantable pacer systems with transvenous leads became popular among specially trained medical cardiologists because the procedure required minimal surgery. By positioning electrodes through veins, the technique eliminated the need for an open-chest procedure in which pacer electrodes would be sutured directly on the heart. Because technologically inferior transvenous leads had an early history of displacement, migration and perforation,[11] Zoll adamantly maintained that a lead solidly secured to the outer surface of the heart by suture or other means was preferable to a transvenous electrode that was passively attached to the inner wall of a heart chamber.

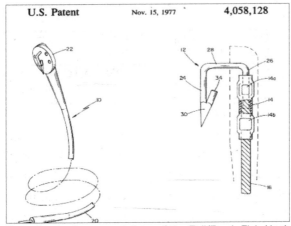

U.S. Patent	Nov. 15, 1977	4,058,128

Two of several representations of the Zoll/Frank Fish Hook Electrode from their patent.

To counter the popularity of long-term transvenous lead placement in "permanent" pacemaker systems, Drs. Paul Zoll and Howard Frank dramatically changed their traditional open-chest approach, inventing a "fish hook" sutureless lead that was introduced through a limited incision below the breastbone. The "hook" could be imbedded in either the right atrium or ventricle by a push or a pull. The electrode was ideal for both adults and children. It was especially well suited to the latter's thin heart wall. Zoll and Frank presented the new concept to the Medtronic Corporation in 1975 and asked the company to consider a collaboration. Zoll and Frank's application for a patent on August 26, 1976, was granted on November 15, 1977, and assigned number 4058128. (See figure this page.) Five years later, Medtronic modified and marketed the fish hook pacemaker lead as models 4951 and 4951M. Neither model ever experienced a defect requiring a safety advisory or a recall. Zoll and Frank were the innovators and the first to prove that a fish hook electrode was feasible. They are responsible for the benefits derived from its limited, sub-breastbone approach that permitted placement under direct vision, avoided an open-chest operation, and hastened patient recovery.[12,13,14]

Emergency Management Of Slow Heart Rate

In the late 1960s and early 1970s, emergency transvenous pacing was rapidly changing the practice of those physicians engaged in acute care. Zoll's objections to transvenous pacing were an expanded version of those raised in 1959 when he consulted on Pinkus Shapiro, the index patient of Seymour Furman and John Schwedel in New York.[15] Paul Zoll believed that emergency management of a barely beating or non-beating heart with a hastily placed temporary transvenous pacing electrode was ill advised and unacceptable for several reasons. By necessity, cardiac stimulation would be delayed to render the operative field sterile and by the need to advance the pacing electrode blindly through a potentially tortuous venous route to the proper heart chamber. Once in place, the electrode could displace, cause arrhythmias, or perforate through the muscular wall of the chamber. The procedure also carried an inherent risk of introducing systemic infection. But Zoll also recognized that the major objection to his 1952 closed-chest transthoracic pacemaker was its pain-producing electric shocks.

Zoll's approach to a viable correction of heart block, or an otherwise inadequate heart rate that required emergency care, came in two stages. The first was to collaborate with Arthur Linenthal in developing emergency protocols to increase heart rate with dilute solutions of isoproterenol or epinephrine, which are potent heart-rate stimulating medications. Continuous infusion of either often aroused the heart to beat at a constant, satisfactory rate until the patient promptly recovered. If the medications were effective, and the patient dependent upon them, a temporary or long-term pacemaker would be placed under ideal sterile conditions.[16-19] The second phase was the early 1980s reinvention of the closed-chest pacemaker as a significant and tolerable life-saving instrument.[20] That discovery will be detailed in Chapter 18.

Other Ventures

Paul Zoll's close-knit group of subterranean Laboratory KB-6 collaborators ventured beyond modifying old ideas. Supported by a grant from the Radio Corporation of America, more commonly known as RCA, the team wrestled with microwave heating, focused on selective areas of the heart, to increase rate. The effort ended in failure.[21,22]

Another initiative was to apply a chest thump or poke that caused a heart to beat. The research initiative was inspired by an observation that mechanical energy making contact near the heart could elicit a cardiac contraction.[23] Historically the phenomenon had been associated with the rare, undesirable consequence of collapse and sudden death. The problem was termed *Commotio Cordis* by the ancients. Today this tragic misfortune is understood as a cascade of events that starts with a blow to the chest that occurs co-incident with the vulnerable period of the cardiac cycle. The blow elicits an extra beat that triggers ventricular fibrillation and death.[24] Such cases are headlined when chest trauma causes a participant to collapse while engaged in a sport. Paul Zoll reasoned that mechanically induced heart beats could be both beneficial and be safe if the vulnerable period was avoided in those hearts that had an adequate blood supply. People with hearts fueled by an inadequate blood supply, or so-called ischemic hearts, would be excluded from consideration. He conjectured that sequential thumps could keep an electrically silent heart beating and a properly timed thump might terminate some forms of rapid heart action, returning the heart to a stable rhythm. It was Bernard Lown who likely made one of the earliest observations of a chest blow that terminated rapid heart action. The serendipitous event occurred in his animal laboratory at the Harvard School of Public Health in the late 1960s. Lown coined the term *thumpversion* to describe it.[25]

An anecdote is told about a patient with dizzy spells who had a heart rhythm recorder in place when he passed out while driving an automobile, hit a tree, struck his chest on the automobile steering column and immediately woke up. The recorder revealed that he had passed out due to rapid ventricular tachycardia that terminated when his chest collided with the steering column. To electively reproduce that lucky accidental outcome, Paul Zoll started to develop a chest thumper that could be synchronized to strike during the safe period of the cardiac cycle. He proposed this innovation for therapeutic application and to provide experimental insights into cardiac muscle mechanics. After years of effort, the chest thumper remained unfinished, until an engineer/patient of Paul Zoll offered to redesign an unsatisfactory version of the thumper in 1976. Within a week "from the goodness of his heart" the patient delivered a finished product.[26] The core of the instrument was a modified staple gun, as shown in the picture below. It was used in a number of experiments.[27,28,29]

It is of interest that in the late 1970s, Bernard Lown, at the neighboring Harvard School of Public Health, used the Zoll concept to perform clinical and animal experiments.[30,31] While mechanically thumping the closed-chests of oxygen-starved dogs, Lown's group induced rapid repetitive ventricular responses and speculated that the method might identify patients at risk of sudden death. Chest-thump-induced ventricular tachycardia in a patient would be a marker of underlying ischemic heart disease, as was the case with the dogs in the experimental model. Patients at risk would be treated with antiarrhythmic drugs.[32]

In the last analysis, too many patients complained that an effective thump was uncomfortable, so Paul Zoll withdrew the device from therapeutic consideration. Yet manual chest thump is still used by some rescuers in the initial phase of cardiac resuscitation, and continues to save lives.

While balancing his life-long commitments to family and to improving the health of patients, Paul Zoll made major contributions to medical progress through innovation, research and discovery. During a 20-year span, Zoll was the

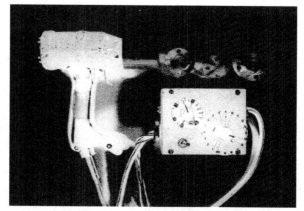

The staple gun is shown on the left, with several sizes of impact discs in the upper right, and the synchronizer control box below them. Negative image ©1976 Massachusetts Medical Society. With permission.

first to closed-chest pace a patient, the first to electrically alarm-monitor a patient for a dangerous heart rhythm, the first to closed-chest defibrillate a patient and the second to implant a long-term, self-contained pacer in a patient. He was also responsible for lesser discoveries such as administration of dilute cardiac accelerants, protocols for emergency management of cardiac arrest, the fish-hook electrode and the "thumper." Along the way, Paul received awards and honors from specialty organizations, which he accepted with grace and humility. After those 20 years of discovery, the time had come for him to receive America's equivalent of the Nobel Prize.

SEVENTEEN

THE LASKER: AMERICA'S EQUIVALENT TO THE NOBEL PRIZE

In 1973, the Albert Lasker Award in Medical Research was shared by Paul Zoll and William Kouwenhoven. The award honors individuals who make significant contributions in clinical and basic research toward understanding and curing diseases that are frequent causes of death and disability. It is administered by the Lasker Foundation, the legacy of Albert Lasker, an entrepreneur and innovator who amassed great wealth by infusing modernity into the advertising industry.

The Lasker was the crowning recognition among the many bestowed upon Dr. Zoll. The award recognized that both Zoll and Kouwenhoven had discovered therapies that restored life to tens of thousands ravaged by cardiovascular disease. The Lasker citation mentions Paul Zoll's contributions to resuscitation with external and implantable cardiac pacing, cardiac monitoring, and external cardiac defibrillation. William Kouwenhoven was honored for his life-long contributions to defibrillation and the discovery of external cardiac massage. Each recipient received a monetary award, a certificate and a statuette of the Winged Victory of Samothrace, otherwise known as the Nike of Samothrace.

Privately, Paul was excited and truly honored to receive a Lasker. Mary Zoll could not recall her father being so animated as when he learned about the impending award. Mary believed that dad was excited because the Lasker was public recognition of the importance of his then 23-year dedication to making life-saving discoveries.[1] But publicly, Paul, in typical fashion, gave no advance

Jeanne Roger's 23 Pacemaker Procedures
1963 through 2000
Epicardial Pacemaker Operations

Date	Duration	System	Features	Comments
1 3/13/63	18 months	Electrodyne	Platinum-plated electrodes VOO	Thorocotomy #1. Sub-pectoralis placement → Infected pacer pocket
2 9/2/64	6 days	Temporary external pacer		Infection with coagulase negative staph albus. Mesh removed. Wires attached to external pacer → sharp rise of thresholds to limits of external pacer
3 9/8/64	11 months	Electrodyne	VOO	Thorocotomy #2. Postero-lateral approach. Abdominal pacer placement. Infection had tracked along electrodes to heart. Loose wire removed. Other wire clipped. (42 months later recurrent staph albus coagulase negative infection at same site) → pacer system failure
4 8/27/65	8 months			Syncope. Wire failure. System unipolarized → Pacer system failure
5 4/7/66	1 month			Fractured ground wire. Replaced → Pacer system failure
6 5/12/66	1 month		Medical management	Both wires failed. Generator removed. Wires clipped. Returned to medical floor in idioventricular rhythm to await implant of advanced pacer system
7 5/15/66	4 months	Electrodyne	Bentov plug-in system Bentov electrodes VOO	Thorocotomy #3. Rectopectoral placement → intermittent system failure
8 9/12/66	1 month			Plug failure. Replace plug. Unipolarize system → system failure
9 10/13/66	4 months			Both plugs faulty. Replace Bentov plugs and extra-thoracic electrodes. Resume bi-polar pacing → intermittent failure and diaphragmatic twitch
10 2/11/67	9 months	Electrodyne	VOO	One faulty electrode responsible for twitch. Pacer replaced. System unipolarized → intermittent system failure
11 11/12/67	4 months	Electrodyne H style	High-output 7.0 volts VOO	Ground wire migrated. New generator, ground wire and plug → system failure
12 3/15/68	12 days	Electrodyne H style	High-output VOO	Wire break within plug. Replace plug and proximal wire. New generator. Infected pocket of fluid noted about wire placed in 1963 and clipped in procedure 3, 9/8/64. The organism isolated had same characteristics → system failure

notice of the award to his friends or relatives. According to cousin Elliot Mahler, they learned from the media after the fact. "Then, the news spread like wild fire. Paul shunned publicity. He wanted nothing to do with center stage."[2]

The award ceremony was held at the St. Regis Hotel in New York City on November 14, 1973. Paul's wife, Janet, and several of his closest colleagues attended. Because Paul always measured his triumphs in human terms, he asked Jeanne Rogers, a long-term patient, to also be his guest. It was unlikely that he set a precedent by attending an honors ceremony with a patient. Wilson Greatbatch, who engineered the first fully contained implantable pacemaker, recalled that "an older woman," who had been treated with one of his

Jeanne Rogers' 23 Pacemaker Procedures
1963 through 2000

(Continued from previous page)

Date	Duration	System	Features	Comments
13 3/27/68	14 months			Syncope. Slow pulse. Faulty ground plug. Plug and wire replaced → system failure
14 6/9/70	6 months	Electrodyne H style	High-output 7.0 volts VOO	High threshold electrode. Pacer replaced → system failure
15 12/16/70	3 days	Electrodyne H style	High-output 7.0 volts VOO	High threshold centrally at heart. Replace generator and extrathoracic electrode → intermittent system failure
12/19/70	8 days		Medical management	Decision to abandon epicardial system. Arrange for endocardial system

Endocardial Pacemaker Operations

Date	Duration	System	Features	Comments
16 12/27/70	22 months	Cordis 1167-95	Single-rate VVI mercury zinc batteries	Right-sided system → rate slowing
17 10/17/72	11 months	Cordis Ventricor	Single-rate VVI mercury zinc batteries	Elective pacer replacement → system failure. Premature battery depletion
18 9/6/73	28 months	Medtronic 5931	Variable pulsewidth VVI mercury zinc batteries	Pacer replacement → rate slowing
19 1/23/76	99 months	Medtronic Spectrax 5985	Multi-programmable VVI lithium battery	Pacer replacement → system failure. High threshold lead after 13 years or service
20 4/12/84	102 months	Cordis 233F Sequecor	DDD. lithium battery	Dual chamber. New unipolar electrodes → rate slowing
21 9/13/85				Remove Medtronic Spectrax generator from right chest. Cap and abandon lead
22 10/14/92	97 months	Medtronic Elite 7075	DDD. lithium battery	Generator replacement → rate slowing
23 11/8/00	18 months	Medtronic Sigma SDR 3064	DDD. lithium battery	Generator replacement

Epicardial=open-chest procedure; lead(s) placed from surface of heart. Endocardial=closed-chest procedure; lead(s) placed from transvenous approach to inner surface of heart. VOO=ventricular pacing without sensing, thus continuous uninterrupted pacing. VVI=ventricular pacing with sensing and response to sensing; permits on-demand pacing and avoids vulnerable period. DDD=dual chamber (atrium and ventricle) pacing, each chamber sensing and responding to sensing.

pacemakers, accompanied him to an award dinner when he was designated Engineer of the Year by his professional society. The media referred to the woman as "the pacemaker queen."[3]

Mrs. Rogers was living proof of the ultimate success of Paul's mission to spare the lives of the unfortunate who suffer from Stokes-Adams attacks. Born with complete heart block, as a child Jeanne suffered from brief fainting spells. After a cardiac arrest during an appendectomy at age seven, she was referred to Dr. Alexander Nadas of Children's Hospital, Boston.[4] Nadas, a cardiologist, continued to follow Jeanne into adulthood while she attempted to have a normal lifestyle. In 1959 she met Robert Rogers, an automobile mechanic who later would operate his own repair shop. When they married the following year, the couple was advised not to have children. But during a routine office visit, Dr. Nadas learned that Jeanne was pregnant. He immediately called Dr. Zoll, saying, "I have a couple of kids here that need your help. Take it easy on them."[5] Zoll saw them the same day and arranged for Jeanne to be followed in the pregnancy clinic by Dr. Dupont, an obstetrician. The couple met with Drs. Dupont and Zoll weekly until baby Bobbie was born on July 3, 1962. Thereafter, Jeanne's frequent and severe syncopal attacks prompted Dr. Zoll to recommend an implantable pacemaker. Mrs. Rogers was receptive to the idea after learning that a pacemaker would allow her to safely enlarge her family. Drs. Howard Frank and Paul Zoll placed an Electrodyne pacer system on March 13, 1963. Mrs. Rogers subsequently had two daughters. She is the world's first pacemaker patient to give birth. Her refusal to be in the Guinness Book of World Records was emphatically supported by Dr. Zoll.

As an early recipients in Paul's series of long-term pacemaker patients, Jeanne Rogers represents the evolution of the implantable pacemaker (see table on previous two pages). She experienced all the trials, tribulations and uncertainties of those early unreliable devices, which Zoll reflected on in his Lasker presentation. He told how managing pacer patients was a nightmare of lead failure or breakage, premature battery failure and frequent component failure.[6] In addition to all of those complications, Mrs Rogers endured pacemaker replacements and infection without complaint. She exhibited total confidence that all would be well, because Dr. Zoll always appeared to be calm and unconcerned. "If he wasn't concerned, why should I be anxious?"[7]

Mrs. Rogers recalled the Lasker ceremony 30 years after the event. She described the ball-room at the St. Regis Hotel as beautiful. Approximately 250 guests attended. Dr. Michael DeBakey was master of ceremonies and made the presentations. Paul's wife, Janet, insisted that Jeanne sit with Paul at the head table where Dr. DeBakey and William Kouwenhoven also sat. In addition to sitting with the dignitaries through the program, Jean also stood with them at the podium.

Because the Lasker was presented during a luncheon ceremony, Janet and Paul had packed their luggage before the presentation for a return flight to Boston the same day. Without storage room to transport his award, Paul

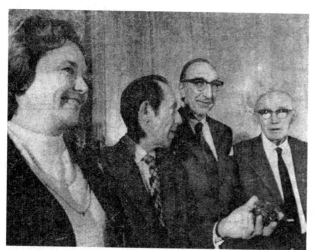

A photograph reproduced from a newspaper shows Jeanne Rogers and Paul Zoll at the Lasker Awards. From left, Rogers, Zoll, Michael DeBakey and William Kouwenhoven. By Mel Finkelstein. © Daily News LP, New York. With permission.

entrusted Jeanne to return to Boston with his Winged Victory of Samothrace.[8] The gesture seemed to distinguish Jeanne as Paul's "pacemaker queen," in the same sense as the patient of Dr. Wilson Greatbatch who had accompanied him to his award ceremony. It also reflected the close friendship that was by then well established between Jeanne Rogers, Paul Zoll, and their families.

The friendship developed during the dozen years that preceded the award in 1973, beginning when Jeanne first became a cardiac patient of Dr Zoll. It continued after the award. Ross Zoll learned automotive mechanics in Robert's repair shop during a summer vacation from school.[9] Each family made house calls. Bob went to Paul's home with Jeanne when there was need to have Dr. Zoll review one of her complaints, and he sometimes came alone to correct an automotive problem on Paul's car. Of course, Paul also made house calls when Jeanne was not well.

After Paul returned to his routine at Beth Israel Hospital following the Lasker, Herman Blumgart and Paul's close colleagues – accustomed to Paul's predilection to shun publicity – sent him an invitation to attend a Lasker celebration in their own honor, even though they were hosting it themselves.[10] They hoped that Paul would attend as a guest, knowing that he would refuse if the celebration was in his honor.

At the time that Paul received the Lasker, 23 of 47 former recipients had already gone on to win a Nobel Prize.[11] Paul never spoke of becoming a Nobel laureate, but Janet often mentioned that he deserved it.[12] When a patient congratulated him on the Lasker and suggested that he might receive a future

Nobel, Paul's written reply brushed aside the speculation as a sign of "soft-heartedness and soft-headedness."[13] Friends and colleagues who believed that political and personal maneuvering influenced a Nobel invitation, predicted that Paul would not be so honored. A close family friend of the Zolls remembered her father's forecast that there wouldn't be a Nobel in Paul's future because "He didn't have a political bone in his body...and would not be able to put together the kind of campaign that is required of candidates to promote themselves into the Nobel."[14] In 1992, Robert Goldwyn, Clinical Professor of Surgery at Harvard Medical School, suggested that Paul Zoll be considered for a Nobel Prize. Nomination papers were drawn up for the 1993 award. Then the trail to Stockholm abruptly ended without explanation.[15]

When Paul Zoll received the Lasker, the foundation cited his developing four separate discoveries. Each resulted in a paradigm shift in cardiac care. They were the closed-chest defibrillator, the clinical cardiac monitor, the external closed-chest pacemaker and the life-saving, life-normalizing, long-term implantable pacemaker. With emphasis on the long-term implantable pacemaker, the citation stated with somewhat ungrounded enthusiasm that "pacemakers... are Paul Zoll's invention."[16] Eighteen years later, when Dwight Harken asked Paul about his wishes for self-remembrance, Paul listed only three of his discoveries that had been mentioned in the Lasker citation. He enigmatically omitted his development of the world's second fully implanted, self contained pacemaker that had been placed in Michael Seiffer.[17] Was the omission an oversight on Paul's part? Was it because he was not the first to succeed, only wanting to be remembered for his three firsts (closed-chest pacing, alarmed cardiac monitors and closed-chest defibrillation)? Was the reason because Michael Seiffer had a suboptimal result? Or was it because the road to success was long and interrupted by many frustrating failures? The answer is unknown.

Jeanne Rogers experienced the frequent complications that were common among the early pacer implant patients. Carl Orecklin's course offers another vivid example of the problems that tormented the early pioneering doctors and their patients. Orecklin, a public school teacher in Michigan, suffered from acquired heart block at age 26 when his heart was permanently damaged by viral myocarditis, an infection that causes inflammation of the heart. In 1963, doctors in Detroit implanted a General Electric pacemaker. During the

Carl Orecklin's 16 Pacemaker Procedures
1963 through 2000

Epicardial Pacemaker Operations

	Date	Duration	System	Features	Comments
1	6/28/63	4 months	General Electric	Sub-cutaneous coil for rate control	Thorocotomy #1. Failed early. Sub-costal abdominal generator placement. Hemothorax. Transfusions. Hepatitis C
2	10/19/63	3 months	General Electric	VOO	→ failed early. Intermittent capture. Hemopericardium
3	1/21/64	23 months	Electrodyne New wires	VOO	Thorocotomy #2. Left posterior approach. Generator under pectoralis muscle. Battery depletion
4	12/8/66	8 months	Electrodyne I	VOO	→ Sudden slowing. Faulty plug
5	8/17/67	6 months	Electrodyne I	VOO	→ Intermittent pacing. Wire fracture
6	5/12/68	6 months	Electrodyne I	VOO	System unipolarized → Intermittent capture
7	12/25/68	7 months	Electrodyne I	VOO	→ intermittent capture, unclear reasons. New system required
8	7/8/69	11 months	Electrodyne I New wires	VOO	Thorocotomy #3 → Wire fracture
9	6/23/70	24 months	Electrodyne I	VOO	System unipolarized → System failure. Presumed battery depletion corroborated. New generator placed at procedure #10
10	6/29/72	1 day	Electrodyne I	VOO	New generator → system failure in hours
11	6/30/72	3 months			Generator #10 retained. Ground wire, plugs, extra-thoracic electrode replaced → failure

Endocardial Pacemaker Operations

	Date	Duration	System	Features	Comments
12	9/18/72	32 months	Cordis pacer and lead	VOO	Transvenous endocardial system. Absent cephalic vein. Right external jugular vein. Unipolar system → Elective replacement
13	5/20/75	39 months	Medtronic 5931	Variable pulsewidth VOO	Lead adapter needed → Battery depletion
14	5/28/78	131 months	Medtronic 5973	Multi-pro-grammable VVI	Lithium battery → Battery depletion
15	7/26/89	128 months	Medtronic 8423	Multi-pro-grammable VVI	→ Elective replacement. Concern regarding 28-year-old Cordis lead
16	3/14/00		Medtronic Sigma 303 New generator and lead	Multi-pro-grammable VVIR	Threshold too high on Cordis lead. Thus new system placed. Rate-responsive system more physiological. Steroid elution electrode tip. Bipolar system

Epicardial=open-chest procedure; lead(s) placed from surface of heart. Endocardial=closed-chest procedure; lead(s) placed from transvenous approach to inner surface of heart. VOO=ventricular pacing without sensing, thus continuous uninterrupted pacing. VVI=ventricular pacing with sensing and response to sensing; permits on-demand pacing and avoids vulnerable period. DDD=dual chamber (atrium and ventricle) pacing, each chamber sensing and responding to sensing.

operation, Carl bled into his left chest. After the procedure, the pacemaker site became infected. Three months later, the pacemaker failed, was replaced, and later removed because of unresolved infection. On the recommendation of local doctors, Orecklin was transferred to the care of Dr. Samuel Levine at Boston's Peter Bent Brigham Hospital. After failing a trial of rate accelerating medications, Levine asked Paul Zoll to consult. Zoll arranged a transfer to Beth Israel Hospital, eliminated the infection and had Dr. Howard Frank perform a second open-chest procedure to release adhesions binding the lung to the chest wall and to implant a new Electrodyne pacer system. Carl was restored to a normal lifestyle. From then on, he returned to Boston's Beth Israel Hospital whenever his pacemaker failed. Once, with a fuzzy head from a heartbeat of less than 20 per minute, Carl had a friend drive him to the airport. Carl took a plane to Boston, reluctantly passed up the in-flight meal, and arrived intact to once again place himself under the care of his saviors, Paul Zoll and Howard Frank.[18] Carl Orecklin's perils under their guidance are charted in the table on the preceding page. He died from a weak heart at the age of 72. During 46 of those years, Carl was sustained by implanted pacemakers.

For recipients like Jeanne Rogers and Carl Orecklin, electrodes were the Achilles heel of their pacemaker systems and all types of electrodes continue to be a problem. Manufacturer recalls and advisories currently involve thousands of lead implants.[19,20] In one noteworthy case, Edward Giberti suffered 22 unnecessary internal defibrillator shocks during a 48-hour period because of an implanted defibrillator electrode fracture. After correction, he had to cope with acute traumatic stress syndrome.[21]

From the outset of his journey in device development, Paul Zoll searched for the Holy Grail of a reliable electrode. In 1963, when his search led to the Simplex Wire Company with a request for a thin wire electrode that could flex 36,792,000 times each year for 50 years, he was seeking a solution for a young woman pacemaker patient who he hoped would live at least another 50 years.[22] That patient was Jeanne Rogers. Her adult life-long course with an implanted pacemaker fulfilled Paul's expectations. No wonder when asked about Paul Zoll some 43 years after her first implant, she answered, "He was not only my doctor, he was my angel."[23]

EIGHTEEN

RETURN TO BASICS
THE LAST OF THE RESEARCH PROJECTS

Brushed aside by the forces of change, transthoracic pacing lay dormant for at least two decades while the preferred method became point-of-care emergency transvenous pacing in the field. The "game changer" was driven by advanced design pacing catheters that could be positioned without x-ray guidance. But Paul Zoll remained steadfast in opposition to this approach because of the amount of time it required. He believed that many victims of asystolic cardiac arrest died or suffered unnecessary irreparable damage because of delayed cardiac reactivation that could have been averted by immediate transthoracic cardiac pacing.[1] While Zoll's appeals fell on deaf ears, he continued to pursue his laboratory research. After distant microwave heart warming trials failed to increase surgically induced slow heart rates in animals during 1976 and 1977,[2,3] Paul and his collaborators met to develop a new initiative. During a planning session, Alan Belgard rose from his chair, walked to the chalkboard and boldly wrote "Painless External Electrical Pacing."[4] The most critical word was *painless.*

The original 1952 external pacemaker had been reconfigured several times. Its size was minimized, battery power was added, and in one model a monitor and defibrillator were combined into a multipurpose emergency unit. However, despite such improvements patient pain remained a formidable barrier to emergency transthoracic pacing. Painless, or near painless pacing would be a technological and therapeutic breakthrough to justify Paul Zoll's tenacious faith in the method.

Pacing pain is caused by forceful skeletal muscle contractions and nerve receptor stimulation. When Paul Zoll started the re-invention initiative, Alan Belgard, Electrodyne, and most other manufacturers used two-inch diameter metal discs as electrodes, which concentrated all of the pacemaker's stimulus energy onto a small surface. As one possible remedy for pacer-induced pain, Alan Belgard suggested abandoning small metallic disc electrodes in favor of large sponge-like cloth conductive pads that could adhere to a contoured chest.[5] The larger diameter, non-metallic, high impedance contacts with skin would diffuse the electrical current density energy as a means of reducing pain.

A second theory for reducing pain was to deliver a constant low current during a longer interval than the prevailing two milliseconds standard of that time. Paul Zoll believed that the optimal stimulus delivery time was known, confirmed, "set in stone" and that its lengthening would be hazardous.[6] But Ross Zoll, a, credentialed physicist, was less certain and argued the point with his father. So Ross proposed a series of experiments to resolve the dispute. The result: a longer delivery time between five and 40 milliseconds was effective, safe, and incrementally reduced pain as delivery time increased.

The investigators cobbled together a system that included each element: constant electrical current, increased delivery time and large, sponge-like electrodes. To validate the concept, each think-tank member self-experimented with the pacemaker while a defibrillator was on standby in case an errant electrical stimulus induced a hazardous ventricular arrhythmia.[7] It is unclear if self-testing was solely to prove the successful conclusion of their deliberations or if the group members were also adhering to the fifth principle of the Nuremberg Code, "No human shall be the subject of a medical experiment that has the potential of disability or death unless the investigator undergoes the procedure."[8] The discomfort level among Zoll's team ranged from "painless" to "tolerable". However, during later extensive clinical testing, some outliers experienced excessive pain.[9]

In the privacy of his medical-office examining room, Paul Zoll mentioned the new pacemaker re-invention to Edmund "Leigh" Stein, who prior to becoming a long-term patient himself, first met Paul when Leigh accompanied his physician-father to Paul's office. Leigh appears to have inherited his father's humanity, but he did not pursue a medical career. His preferred course was

Harvard Business School, then the presidency and chief executive officer of a packaging company. His entrepreneurial experience prompted him to make the delicate suggestion that Paul create a business to showcase the new invention.[10] Paul resisted. He had either avoided financial gain from past electrotherapeutic inventions or it had avoided him. Stein eventually realized that Paul's major impediment to developing a business plan, obtaining a patent and raising capital was his disinterest in such matters and general dislike for lawyers. With persuasive persistence, Stein wore Zoll down until he reluctantly agreed to a preliminary meeting with a lawyer of Leigh's choice.

Stein's goal was to engage a lawyer who balanced the qualities of superior knowledge and a non-intimidating personality. Leigh arranged a meeting attended by himself, Paul Zoll, who was only 62 inches tall, and a lawyer who was equally short in stature, soft spoken and parsimonious when conversing. During the hour-long session, Paul and the lawyer exchanged no more than a few sentences. Unwilling to interrupt the silence, Stein did not speak.[11] The meeting was a great success. Paul liked the lawyer and moved ahead with establishing the business in 1980.

After the two Zolls and Alan Belgard secured a patent on September 14, 1982, Paul considered selling or licensing the rights to the invention because he felt that implementing the business plan would cause too great a distraction from his ongoing research. With that aim in mind, Stein and Zoll traveled to Washington State to investigate those possibilities with an established medical technology company. When the company made an insulting, extremely low, near-nothing offer for the patent, Paul decided to stay the course.

The next phase of business formation was to capitalize the startup. Leigh gathered a few associates to consider investing in the nascent company. The group of high- powered businessmen met in Paul Zoll's untidy basement laboratory for a demonstration. Leigh Stein was the sole volunteer among the group to experience transthoracic pacing.[12] The meeting was similar to the one described by Thomas Claflin II, a venture capital investor who recalled a demonstration of the new device in which Ross Zoll was paced by Paul.[13] In the first meeting, the painless pacemaker's potential to survive in the marketplace impressed Stein's group. The investors opened their wallets. Modest Paul refused to have the company named after himself. Instead it initially bore the title Ross Research after his son.

When the company grew, its next identity was ZMI, (a cryptic acronym for Zoll Medical Instruments Incorporated). Paul enjoyed his role on the board of directors, remaining within his area of expertise by serving as an adviser to an expanding staff of medical electronic engineers. Paul constantly emphasized the need to be uncompromising on safety standards. As word spread through the medical community about the painless external pacemaker, then undergoing clinical trials, Paul responded to an urgent request to use his pacer on a needy patient at Boston City Hospital (BCH). The result was impressive. In the afterglow, Rodney Falk, the lead BCH cardiologist asked that his hospital be a test center for the new device. Paul agreed, but insisted that the sponge electrodes be moistened with City of Boston tap water, which provided a higher impedance – or greater electrical resistance, a key to minimizing pain – than Cambridge City tap water.[14] In close collaboration with Dr. Zoll, the study was completed, was favorable and was published in 1983.[15]

Other clinical investigators, who were approved by ZMI to use the new non-invasive temporary pacemaker, received S.O.S. calls to help patients in special circumstances. One such patient at Children's Hospital Boston suffered with malignancy, nausea, vomiting and syncope. A transvenous temporary pacemaker was contraindicated because bone marrow depression posed a dual threat of infection and bleeding. Instead, the patient had a ZMI pacer in place for a month in anticipation of a prolonged syncopal attack.[16,17] Meanwhile, other institutions organized studies that confirmed, with some exceptions, that the pacemaker was effective and well tolerated. To advance within the industry, the company had to expand its reach and product line. There was another infusion of venture capital, Food and Drug Administration approval for ZMI to market its new non-invasive temporary pacemaker (NITP), and a change in leadership with Rolf Stutz replacing Leigh Stein as President of ZMI in July 1983, with Leigh becoming a member of the board of directors. Leigh, a man of many accomplishments, regarded his role of creating and leading the company through its infancy as the most gratifying period of his illustrious career.[18]

In 1984, evidence suggested that three medical device companies had likely infringed on the ZMI pacemaker patent. When ZMI sought legal redress, Paul

Zoll was asked to testify in the role of a key witness. Rolf Stutz recalled that Paul was usually calm, precise, disinterested, and very detached. On one occasion, however, when an aggressive opposing lawyer impugned Paul's integrity, he came alive, bristled, eyes narrowed and his testimony destroyed the lawyer.[19]

Bowing to repeated requests, in 1992 Paul agreed that the company name be changed to Zoll Medical. The corporation evolved into an industry leader in resuscitation with products that happily coincided with Paul Zoll's unswerving medical mission.

The name Zoll is synonymous with the Zoll box (original transthoracic pacemaker); a Zoll (defined by hospital trainees as a "unit of resistance" to describe Paul ignoring their clinical recommendations) and the Zoll Medical Corporation that, at the time of his death, had equipment inscribed with the name *Zoll* assisting in 1,000 resuscitations each day.[20]

Going back to the start of his original research in the early 1950s, Paul Zoll's index pacing concept was to stimulate the heart with an electrode in the esophagus and another on the front of the chest. In 1983, during one self-test trial with his re-invented "painless" non-invasive temporary pacemaker, Zoll paced his own heart with an esophageal bipolar electrode in the presence of Alan Belgard and a standby defibrillator. His meticulous notes recorded minor subjective discomfort and objective success in sustaining continuous atrial pacing. Zoll concluded that the procedure had promise but needed fine tuning.[21]

That test – seeking to expand the safe usage of his re-invented pacemaker for atrial pacing – pointed to Paul Zoll's last foray in clinical research. In 1989 he was asked by Dr. Warren Manning at Beth Israel Deaconess Medical Center to collaborate in the planning of an esophageal pacing study of the atrial heart chambers. The protocol was to compare conventional, chemical-induced cardiac stress measured by computerized tomography imaging with unproven, rapid esophageal *atrial-chamber*-pacing cardiac stress measured by echocardiogram imaging. Both chemical induced cardiac stress and large chamber pacing methods were known to diagnose a regional lack of heart muscle oxygen, which is a validated surrogate for a critically narrowed coronary artery. In preparation for the study, Warren and Paul self-tested the esophageal pacing portion of the protocol without incident.[22] Although the study was never finished, it completed a circle that encompassed Paul's approximately 40-year career of investigation using almost the same technique that he had explored at its embarkation.

NINETEEN

THE LEGACY
EPILOGUE TO THE PAUL ZOLL STORY

In the winter of his years, Paul Zoll retired from clinical practice. When a close colleague suggested that Paul continue to conduct experiments in the laboratory, he answered, "No, it was the patients, always the patients that powered the research."[1] When his cousin, Elliot Mahler asked, "Do you have any regrets?" Paul answered, "I did so little…there is so much more I should have done."[2]

In the context of that conversation, although his work was unfinished: his impact would be unending.

Paul Zoll retired in 1993 and died from pneumonia on January 5, 1999. The unrelenting progress in electrical suppression of life threatening arrhythmias might have advanced at a much slower pace had Paul died from his first episode of pneumonia on Sitka Island during World War II.

Growing numbers of later day investigators are intent on reducing worldwide arrhythmic deaths, confronting an annual death toll that remains as high as an estimated 450,000 lost lives annually in the U.S.A. alone.[3] The research format for new therapies has dramatically changed from that followed by Paul Zoll during most of his career. Current investigations require collaboration among multiple disciplines within the same institution, hundreds or thousands of subjects, multiple institutions – at times with an international registry. Funding for these studies requires major commitments from government, industry or private philanthropy. Some senior investigators have limited, minimal or no patient responsibilities. Some grind out publications by the score from an institutional headquarters where they strategize and coordinate far flung efforts.

Paul influenced the direction of cardiac therapy while he filled his 18-20 waking hours devoted to work, family and a limited number of friends.[4] Applying his broad vision and a laser focus for detail, Paul approached research projects from the perspective of the challenge he faced from unsolved patient problems. He often approached hazardous arrhythmias with closed-chest electrical therapy, which was Paul's proven point of entry for therapeutic success; success with those methods created a world-wide paradigm shift towards his point of view.

He remained committed to closed chest techniques because they had stood the test of time and they worked well in his hands. Paul Zoll was more interested in patient safety at any cost than the cost effectiveness of a device or a treatment.[5,6] He was more interested in his patient's welfare than personal advancement or financial gain. To many, he appeared to be rigid, reactionary and unaccepting of change. But rather than a weakness, his unwavering commitment was an important constituent of strength. It stemmed from unflagging faith in his methods, unwillingness to readily accept or be distracted by new ideas simply for their novelty, and an ability to refine, re-invent, or newly invent a device to support his wide-angle view of arrhythmic death-threats and their therapies.

Paul's vision and style demanded that he lead a band of colleagues that believed in his mission. They bonded in purpose and in mutual loyalty. He led by indefatigable example, commitment, and a long work day with little need for sleep. Paul Zoll had an infectious optimism for a solution to each patient or research problem confronted in the trenches of the hospital wards or in the research laboratory. Although Paul worked and lived long enough to fulfill his primary mission, he believed that he should have done more, that his work was unfinished. Consistent with his modesty, Zoll did not realize that his footprint will be everlasting.

Because there are pervasive new models of medical practice and research by committee, there may never be another pioneer like Paul Zoll.

APPENDIX ONE

A BRIEF HISTORY OF REANIMATION BY ELECTRIC SHOCK · TO *JUMPSTART* THE HEART

Paul Zoll was aware of historic reports claiming benefit from shocking the chest of the apparent dead. A few early examples are noteworthy.

In 1778, Charles Kite, an English physician, published an essay on the recovery of the apparent dead in which he advocated applying an electrostatic charge across the chest. Kite developed a machine that had a capacitor to store energy, a variable output and two electrodes that could be positioned anywhere on the body.[1] His membership in the London Humane Society, a multinational organization dedicated to reviving victims of drowning and other life-threatening circumstances, gave him access to the society's archival case reports. He came upon that of Catherine Sophie Greenhill, a three-year-old girl, who appeared dead after falling from a second-story window in 1774. A Dr. Squires arrived 20 minutes later and attempted revival with electrical shocks about her body and through her chest until he felt a weak pulse and noted resumption of respirations.[2,3] After remaining comatose for four days, she rapidly recovered. Kite speculated that the youngster most likely had been in coma or suspended animation the entire time, rather than returning from the dead after she had received multiple electric shocks.

A cluster of keen minds that independently arrive at a new idea and hold it in common is a recurring phenomenon that accelerates progress. That happened with Mark Lidwell and Albert Hyman in the late 1920s. Without personal contact and continents apart, each seized upon the idea of directly stimulating the heart with a plunge-needle electrode.

In 1927, Albert Hyman started preliminary work on his pacemaker in New York City. He was making progress when Mark Lidwell, an Australian anesthetist, presented details of a pacemaker apparatus to his colleagues at the Medical Congress of Australia meeting in 1929. The new invention was portable and powered by line current. It was designed to stimulate an arrested heart via a unipolar needle electrode fashioned with an insulated shaft and non-insulated tip that was plunged through the chest wall to a heart chamber. The ground electrode, needed to complete the circuit, was placed on the skin.[4,5]

Clinicians rarely have adequate expertise to work independently in the field of medical electronics. They usually partner with a highly skilled engineer. Lidwell credited his collaborator, Major Edgar A. Booth of the Physics Department, University of Sidney, with the pacemaker's technical development. The latest version had a wide energy range between 1.5 and 120 volts–although about 16 volts was found to be adequate–a heart-rate range between 80 and 120 beats per minute, and a reverse polarity switch. Lidwell presented a detailed story of how he and his machine revived a stillborn asystolic baby after ten minutes of effective ventricular pacing.[6] All of Lidwell's schematics and machines are lost to history, a fate shared by many of Lidwell's contemporaries.

While Lidwell was at work in Australia, Dr. Albert Hyman collaborated with electrophysiologists in New York City in an attempt to construct a pacemaker in 1928. Immediately after that, between 1929 and 1932, Albert and his brother Charles, both of New York City, designed three different pacemaker models.[7] The extent of Charles' formal technical training is unclear. Dr. Albert Hyman claimed that each of the three models he and his brother developed was effective in both experimental and clinical trials. Hyman promoted his methods and exaggerated his results to the press. He also spoke of successes in interviews. However, he never published or presented hard data to support the claims. They were later reviewed critically by Seymour Furman, who found them to be without substance.[8] An engineer working for the Siemens Company, which had contracted to manufacture the Hymanotor model, concluded that the pacemaker lacked enough power to stimulate a heart with its electrode needle in proximity to, or directly on, the right atrium. Close scrutiny of Hyman's published electrocardiograms revealed the presence of pacemaker stimuli but showed no excitation of heart muscle.

At a presentation before a select audience of colleagues, Hyman claimed that he had succeeded in pacing a limited number of patients. But the event could not be recalled by anyone on Hyman's list of attendees. Albert Hyman's later claim of success in a limited number of patients with Stokes-Adams disease was rightfully called into question because all were paced from the right atrium, an unphysiological locus that could not rectify the primary problem of blocked electrical transmission between the atrium and ventricle. Albert Hyman scrupulously shunned plunging the pacemaker needle into the ventricle for fear of provoking ventricular fibrillation. He avoided comprehensive reporting of results, breaching a fundamental tenant that serious science must be properly and thoroughly reported for verification.

Investigations by Seymour Furman and associates indicated that the Hyman brothers might have deliberately deceived the public and the medical establishment. The Furman report concluded, "But the fate of their invention, whether it ever resuscitated a human being or even a guinea pig remains a mystery. The current investigation has not turned up new evidence supporting the belief that Hyman invented a workable pacemaker, quite the contrary..." The report ends with an emphatic message, "...investigators and inventors should take from this account a practical lesson: Always keep detailed records of your experimental work and publish or present your results in a timely fashion with full corroborative detail."[9] Unfortunately, historians of pioneering advances in the field of cardiac electronics will not be able to establish primacy for researchers who do not follow Furman's wise advice.

Although they were tainted, Hyman's works and claims of success still deserve a review because of their historic conceptual advances. Albert Hyman published four papers on intracardiac therapy using a conventional needle or electrified needle.[10-13] He also co-authored two medical books.[14,15] Hyman coined the terms "cardiac electrostimulation" and "electronic pacemaker." The Hyman brothers started work on their first pacemaker in 1928 and applied for a patent in 1930, had a working model in 1931, and patent approval in 1933. Images presented in a scientific publication and a popular magazine[16] permitted working reproductions of their first and second models. The third was described in spoken and written accounts without a diagram or photographic likeness. Each pacemaker improved upon its predecessor and each model was named. In sequence, they were "the artificial pacemaker," "the Hymanotor," and "the flashlight pacer" or "life flashlight."

While the Hyman brothers started work on their concept prior to Lidwell's report, both sets of researchers coincidentally believed that the heart could be stimulated via a needle-like electrode thrust through the chest wall to a heart chamber. However, Hyman's bipolar needle improved upon Lidwell's unipolar design and Hyman's first artificial pacemaker derived its energy from mechanical generation rather than from a line source. It was a hand-carried, hand-cranked, 16-pound electromechanical machine. The Hymanotor, his second model, was smaller, could be easily hand carried and also had a spring motor that was "loaded" by hand. Little is known about the flashlight pacemaker except that it was designed to be lightweight, small enough to be placed in a physician's traditional black bag and powered by a battery.

As scientific discovery evolves, new concepts displace old. Paul Zoll's vision and success with non-invasive pacing that began with his moment of discovery in 1952 displaced the need to open the chest or plunge an electrode through the thorax. However, years later, a 1959 technologically superior Atronic Pacemaker plunge-electrode model – designed to have the tip curve backwards to contact the inner heart wall, rather than contact the outer heart surface or remain free within a blood-filled heart chamber – started a brief revival for plunge-electrode use in desperate circumstances. But the electrode still faced the unresolved risk of striking a coronary artery, since all coronary arteries are theoretically on the surface of the heart. That danger probably accounts for the Atronic Pacemaker electrode eventually falling out of favor.

In their heyday, the plunge-needle pacemakers owed much of their popularity to the self- promotion of Albert Hyman. He claimed proof of concept with animal experiments performed at the Witkin Foundation Cardiac Laboratory at New York's 34-bed Beth David Hospital. In conversation with the medical historian Dr. David Schechter, Albert Hyman stated that he had revived 14 of 43 animals with the flashlight pacemaker.[17] He believed that pacemakers should be used clinically only as a last resort in the narrow context of unexpected cardiac arrest during electrocution, asphyxiation or cardiovascular collapse in victims with apparently healthy, non-diseased hearts. Hyman later drifted from this guideline to revive obviously diseased hearts by providing treatment where he perceived the greatest need. He erroneously believed that his electrode worked because the tip provoked a mechanically induced extra beat upon contact with the heart wall and that subsequent low-intensity electrical stimuli were equivalent to sequential pinpricks. Despite his misconception, he was correct in urging swift action in a crisis, a proven principle required for a successful outcome.

Although Albert never detailed his clinical successes in academic circles, in other arenas he spoke of temporarily resurrecting a 45-year-old woman with mitral stenosis who had been pronounced dead.[18] In a 1932 publication, he wrote, "Although the number of patients successfully treated by this method is still very small, a more or less widespread adoption of the method would unquestionably show the validity of the procedure."[19] A 1932 newspaper article cited a presentation by Albert Hyman at the American Medical Association Convention where he reported that the new artificial pacemaker had reanimated a 70-year-old cardiac patient in his home. The pacemaker permitted the man to live 28 extra hours, just enough time to have parting words with his son.[20] In 1935, he told a small medical group that the Hymanotor had kept a man alive for 24 hours. In 1936, Hyman told a reporter from the New York Times that the flashlight pacemaker was successful in two of seven clinical attempts. A 1936 newspaper column headline shouted, "Electric Needle Restarts Heart. Device Used to Revive Many Persons Officially Pronounced Dead".[21] In 1942, Hyman reported in a transcript that he and a colleague paced the right atrium of a 76-year-old naval officer with Stokes-Adams attacks for 30 minutes.[22] The approach could not have succeeded because the cause of the attacks was blocked conduction between the atrium and ventricle. In 1946, Hyman provided Schechter transcripts of three more successes with Stokes-Adams attacks that were also paced from the right atrium. Based on fuzzy evidence, he later claimed primacy for electrotherapeutic management of Stokes-Adams disease.[23] In time, historians would crown Paul Zoll with that laurel wreath.

Interestingly Albert Hyman's mastery at generating publicity caused a backlash. He was frequently targeted by people who believed that his work and mission were immoral and contrary to the will of God.[24] At a later time, Paul Zoll and Earl Bakken would be so charged.

The careers of Albert Hyman and Paul Zoll had other similarities. Both were educated entirely at Harvard. Both attended the college, the medical school and interned at Harvard teaching hospitals. Hyman interned at Boston City; Zoll interned at Beth Israel. At a later time, both practiced at hospitals established by the Jewish community to accommodate the needs of its under-served immigrants. Hyman practiced at New York's Beth David Hospital and Zoll at Boston's Beth Israel Hospital.

But that is where the similarities end. Paul Zoll was not self promoting, had deep humility and always presented meticulously gathered data to support his conclusions.

APPENDIX TWO

MAJOR AWARDS AND HONORS

1944   United States Army Legion of Merit

1967   John Scott Award, City of Philadelphia, Pennsylvania

1968   Eugene Drake Memorial Lecture and Award, Maine Heart Association

1973   First Wenkebach Memorial Lecture, University of Groningen, The Netherlands

1973   Albert Lasker Award for clinical medical research, New York, NY

1974   Man of the Year Award, Boston Latin School, Boston, Massachusetts

1974   Award of Merit of the American Heart Association, New York, NY

1980   Wunsch Family Foundation Award in Biomedical Engineering, Polytechnic Institute of New York University, New York, NY

1981   Texas Heart Institute Medalist and Ray C. Fish Award, Texas Heart Institute, Houston, Texas

1985   Paul Dudley White Award, Massachusetts Heart Association

1989   Pioneer in Cardiac Pacing and Electrophysiology, North American Society of Pacing And Electrophysiology

1990   Cardiostim Society Medal, 7th International Congress, France

1992   Lifetime Achievement Award, American Heart Association, Dallas, Texas

2002   Portrait of Paul Zoll at the Countway Library, Harvard Medical School, Boston, Massachusetts

APPENDIX THREE

THE GIFT THAT KEEPS ON GIVING

Everyone on the planet is a potential victim of a cardiac arrest or a potential rescuer. Chances of survival for anyone who collapses because of arrested heart action is increased by the level of bystander training in emergency life support. Counterfactual to common belief, bystanders are often first responders in an emergency, rather than trained ambulance, police, or firefighter personnel. Rates of survival are outstanding in communities where courses in basic life support are taught to students in the lower- and upper-level grades of community school systems with subsequent life-long refresher courses for all age groups. Seattle, Washington, is probably the safest place in the U.S. to collapse because that city has made citizen emergency life-support training a priority and has coordinated several departments of municipal first responders with its hospital network. In contrast, there are other communities that do not emphasize bystander training or coordination and communication among first responder services, with the grim result that survival is slim for anyone who collapses within their boundaries.

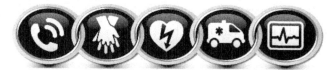

Am. Heart Assn.
With permission.*

The American Heart Association, the American Red Cross, and local public health organizations advocate a five step *Chain Of Survival* emergency response procedure. Each step is a link in the chain, illustrated above.*

The five steps are:

1. Recognize a cardiac arrest and call 911 for an emergency response team.

2. Assess the victim's status regarding consciousness, pulse and respirations. If unconscious and without a pulse, start cardiopulmonary resuscitation with an emphasis on chest compression. Designate someone to search for, and return with, an automated external defibrillator (AED). Rapid chest compression over the lower breast bone must be maintained while the AED leads are attached.

3. Voice prompts from the AED will guide the rescuer through a series of steps. Defibrillation will be requested if indicated.

4. When professionals arrive on the scene, they continue advanced life support during transport to a hospital.

5. Appropriate post cardiac arrest care is determined at the hospital, followed by an individualized plan for diagnostic and therapeutic procedures.

Survival might also hinge on the location of the cardiac arrest. Federal and state mandates require the placement of public-access Automated External Defibrillators–such as the one shown on the facing page–in certain facilities. Designated locations include gaming casinos, airports, health clubs, sport stadiums, airplanes and other locations.

Paul Zoll's discovery of closed-chest cardiac defibrillation in 1955 was his most enduring gift to humanity, which keeps giving with a progression of technical advances such as battery-powered, lightweight portable units with efficient wave forms and other nuances like algorithms for accurate diagnosis of heart rhythm, audio prompts to guide an operator through the resuscitation process including when to defibrillate, and other graphic instructions.

Because modern defibrillators are reasonably priced and affordable by some individuals and institutions, they are often available in non-mandated establishments such as houses of worship, hotels, apartment buildings, social clubs, golf clubs and restaurants. They dot the landscape and are so abundant that advocates prone to wishful thinking are hopeful that emergency AEDs located in see-through wall cabinets will be as abundant as fire alarm boxes.

All physically fit readers should become familiar with the symptoms of a coronary heart attack and those who are living in the U.S. should become certified in basic life support. Contact your local affiliate of the American Heart

Association, American Red Cross, or a public health facility for additional information. Readers living in other countries can identify and contact comparable organizations that are similarly dedicated to saving lives. After instruction, you might be a rescuer who saves a life, and any number of graduates of a life support course might be able to save your life.

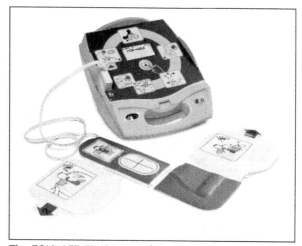

The ZOLL AED PLUS is an advanced model that monitors the rate and depth of chest compressions, records and stores data, advises the operator if defibrillation is required, and incorporates other features. Its size in inches is 5.25 high, 9.50 wide, 11.50 deep. Weight is 6.7 pounds. Courtesy of ZOLL Medical Corporation. With permission.

*Chain Of Survival logo reprinted with permission, 2010 American Heart Association Guidelines for Cardiopulmonary Resuscitation and Emergency Cardiovascular Care, Part 4 CPR Overview, Circulation 2010; 122 {suppl3 }: S676-S684© 2010 American Heart Association, Inc.

GLOSSARY

Alarmed Cardiac Monitor An apparatus that constantly monitors an electro-cardiographic representation of a patient's heart beat. When adjustable rapid or slow rate limits are exceeded, an alarm is triggered. This alerts caregivers to immediately respond.

Antiarrhyhmic A therapy that prevents or corrects an arrhythmia.

Arrhythmia An abnormal heart rhythm that can range from benign to life-threatening.

Aorta The main artery into which the heart pumps blood and from which branches deliver oxygen and nutrients throughout the body.

Asystole Failure of the heart to beat due to absence of an electrical prompt. Also: Absence of electrical or mechanical cardiac activity; Cardiac standstill; Cardiac arrest.

Asynchronous A term that defines a pacemaker that fires at a continuous constant rate without being influenced by surrounding electrical cardiac phenomena.

Automated External Defibrillator (AED) A portable, light weight, battery operated, closed-chest defibrillator that has algorithms to diagnose heart rate and rhythm. Audio prompts instruct an operator when to defibrillate a victim of cardiac arrest.

Bioelectric The electrical phenomena that is common in living tissue.

Cardiac Arrest Failure of the heart to beat or to generate enough power to pump blood. There are two common forms: See Asystole and Ventricular Fibrillation.

Cardiac Monitor See Alarmed Cardiac Monitor.

Cardioversion A word coined by Bernard Lown M.D. to describe the delivery of a direct current therapeutic electric shock to correct a cardiac arrhythmia.

Closed Chest In the context of this book, the term describes a manner in which pacemaker and defibrillator therapy is applied. Electrical stimulation intended for the heart is applied to the external surface of a closed chest, traveling through the chest cavity to reach its target.

Countershock An historic term preferred by Paul Zoll over "Cardioversion" to describe the delivery of an alternating current or direct current electric shock to correct a cardiac arrhythmia.

Coronary Artery A vessel that supplies heart tissue with oxygen and nutrients. There are several named coronary arteries that are responsible for specific areas of the heart.

Defibrillator An apparatus that delivers an electrical shock to correct a fibrillating heart. The shock can be life saving if the condition is ventricular fibrillation. If the condition is atrial fibrillation, return to normal rhythm usually results in diminished symptoms. The apparatus can be for external use intended to deliver a high energy shock to the heart via a closed chest, or at times to deliver a shock directly to the heart in an open-chest procedure, such as at the conclusion of open-chest heart surgery. An internal defibrillator, on the other hand, is implanted within the body, and delivers its shock through bridging electrodes directly to the heart. Alternating or direct current external defibrillators can be powered by wall circuitry. Battery powered or municipal wall circuit powered direct current defibrillators can be synchronized to the "safe period" of the cardiac cycle when treating arrhythmias other than ventricular fibrillation. See Automated External Defibrillator (AED); Cardioversion; Countershock; Synchronize.

Demand Pacing or **(On Demand Pacing)** See Pacemaker.

Electrocardiac Therapy The application of electrical methods to stimulate or deliver a high energy shock to the heart.

Electrocardiogram A graph that represents the electrical forces of the heart's contractions. The graph is generated by an electrocardiograph machine.

Electrode A wire bridge between an electrical power source and the point of delivery. Synonyms used in this book are cardiac electrode, catheter electrode, and wire. There are several electrode configurations depending on the location of the positive and negative poles that are necessary to complete an electrical circuit. They are classified as unipolar, bipolar and multipolar. Catheter electrodes or electrode catheters are placed within veins and guided to the inner surface (endocardium) of a heart chamber. Unipolar or bipolar plunge electrodes were long needles directed through the chest wall to the heart.

Endocardium The inner surface of the heart.

Epicardium The outer surface of the heart.

Heart Block An abnormal heart rhythm that results from some or many of the heart's natural bioelectric pacemaker signals failing to stimulate the main chambers with consequences that vary from a slow heart rate to main chamber ventricular asystole. The condition can be congenital or acquired and is often associated with Stokes-Adams attacks. See Ventricular Septal Defect.

Hypothermia An abnormally low body temperature. A procedure used to preserve organ viability during heart surgery.

Ischemic Inadequate blood flow to an organ with resulting temporary deprivation of oxygen and nutrients.

Jumpstart To correct abruptly. In the context of this book, to abruptly start a non-beating heart with a sequence of electric shocks.

Lesser Arrhythmias Generally refers to non-compromising or compromising, but not life threatening arrhythmias that can be remedied on an elective, non-emergency basis.

Long Term Implantable Pacemaker An implantable and self-sustaining pacemaker that is either fully contained with all of its components or a pacemaker that has a portion of its components implanted within the body and interacts with the remaining portion that is positioned nearby on the surface of the skin. See Pacemaker.

Oscilloscope An instrument with a screen on which is inscribed a continuous image such as an electrocardiogram or other physiological data.

Oxygenated Oxygen laden, as in oxygenated blood

Pacemaker The trigger of stimuli that determines the rate of a sequence of reactions. In other words, the *pace* of a reaction. A pacemaker can be natural as in a biological bioelectric pacemaker, or artificial as in a manufactured pacemaker that delivers a series of electric shocks to stimulate the heart. Varieties of manufactured cardiac pacemakers can stimulate the heart in several ways: through an open chest with bridging electrodes on the outer surface (epicardium) of the heart; through a closed chest; via bridging electrodes or transvenous electrodes from either an external or implanted pacemaker to heart muscle or the inner surface (endocardium) of the heart. Historically there were partially implanted pacemakers that had batteries recharged from a nearby external induction coil, and radiofrequency pacemakers that stimulated the heart from radio waves that were transmitted adjacent to the outer surface of the skin.

The sequence of pacemaker stimuli can be continuous and uninterrupted or it can be *on demand*, occurring only when there is a need to stimulate the heart. See Long Term Implantable Pacemaker.

Prototype An original or first model. Those that follow are copies.

Reset To change. In the context of this book, to convert a life-threatening rhythm into a life-normalizing rhythm by resetting the hazardous rhythm with countershock/cardioversion defibrillation. See Defibrillator.

Rewire To substitute wire electrodes for nature's cardiac conduction system as is the case with pacemakers and implanted pacemaker/defibrillator systems.

Stokes-Adams Attacks (also termed Stokes-Adams Disease) Fainting or near-fainting spells caused by transient or sustained failure of electrical transmission within the heart's conduction system that results in a heart rate that is inadequate to circulate sufficient blood to the brain. See Heart Block.

Synchronize To simultaneously coordinate the occurrence of two events. In the context of this book, to coordinate a direct current cardioversion shock with the safe period of the cardiac electrical cycle while avoiding the unsafe, vulnerable period. Because the delivery of alternating current countershock is prolonged, it could not predictably avoid the vulnerable period. See Vulnerable Period.

Telemetry The process of wireless transmission of information to a receiver. In the context of this book, the transmission of continuous electrical cardiac activity to a distant receiver that records an electrocardiogram of heart rhythm.

Transtelephonic The transmission of continuous electrical cardiac activity via a telephone to a receiver that inscribes the heart rhythm on an electrocardiogram.

Transthoracic The delivery of electrocardiac therapy to the heart through a closed chest. See Pacemaker; Defibrillator.

Transvenous Through veins. In the context of this book, the delivery of electrocardiac therapy to the inner surface of heart chambers (endocardium) via catheter electrodes introduced into veins.

Ventricular Fibrillation A chaotic, continuous, uncoordinated quivering of the heart that renders it incapable of pumping blood.

Ventricular Septal Defect An abnormal communication in the partition that separates the right and left ventricles. The condition is most often congenital and is often labeled a *hole in the heart*. Surgical correction can result in Heart Block.

Vulnerable Period The electrical phase of the cardiac cycle that, if stimulated by an electric shock, mechanical blow, or a spontaneous extrasystole at that time, can result in a sequence of rapid beats that could trigger a life-threatening arrhythmia. See Synchronize.

END NOTES

ONE

1. Zoll PM. The intermediate history of cardiac pacing. In: Harthorn JW, Thalen HJTh, eds. Boston Colloquium on Cardiac Pacing. The Hague-The Netherlands: Martinus Nijhoff Medical Division, 1976: 28

2. Ibid.

3. Schechter DC. Background of clinical cardiac electrostimulation VII. Modern era of artificial cardiac pacemakers. NY State J Med 1972; 73: 1167

4. Zoll PM. The intermediate history of cardiac pacing...Boston Colloquium on Cardiac Pacing...1976: 28

THREE

1. David Kaplan interviewed by Stafford I Cohen February 11, 2011. David is Paul Zoll's first cousin. With permission

2. United States Census Report 1930. Boston, Suffolk Massachusetts. Roll 950; p 12A. The report lists Paul as 18 years old and Herbert as 23 years old. David Kaplan, Mary Zoll and Elsie Zoll spoke of Herbert being four years older than Paul which was accepted because of known inaccuracies in the collection of census data and age differentials that can be misleading.

3. Elsie Zoll interviewed by Stafford I Cohen June 03, 2009. Elsie is Paul Zoll's sister-in-law, Herbert's wife. With permission

4. David Kaplan interviewed by Stafford I Cohen February 11, 2011...With permission

5. Elliot Mahler interviewed by Stafford I Cohen September 09, 2007. Elliot is Paul Zoll's second cousin. With permission

6. Elsie Zoll interviewed by Stafford I Cohen June 03,2009...With permission

7. Cecilia Tucker interviewed by Stafford I Cohen January 21, 2009. Cecilia is Paul Zoll's first cousin, the daughter of Elias. With permission

8. David Kaplan interviewed by Stafford I Cohen February 11, 2011...With permission

9. Ross Zoll PhD MD, interviewed by Stafford I Cohen February 09, 2009. Ross is Paul and Janet's son. With permission

10. Mary Zoll PhD, interviewed by Stafford I Cohen July 26, 2011. Mary is Paul and Janet's daughter. With permission

11. Leona Norman Zarsky MD, interviewed by Stafford I Cohen March 22, 2006. Leona was one of the earliest members of Paul's research team. She was director of the animal experimental laboratory. With permission

12. Alan Belgard BEE, interviewed by Stafford I Cohen February 06, 2007. Alan is Paul's longstanding engineer and collaborator. Together they designed new devices to correct clinical cardiac problems. With permission

13. Cecilia Tucker interviewed by Stafford I Cohen January 21, 2009...With Permission

14. Norman Morris. Ghetto Memories. Growing Up In Dorchester-Roxbury-Mattapan; self published, 2003

15. Norman Morris. Ghetto Memories Revisited. Dorchester-Roxbury-Mattapan As It Was Then, As It Is Now. self published (publication date not stated)

16. David Kaplan interviewed by Stafford I Cohen February 11, 2011...With permission

17. Elsie Zoll interviewed by Stafford I Cohen June 03, 2009...With permission

18. Ross Zoll interviewed by Stafford I Cohen February 09, 2009...With permission

19. Mary Zoll interviewed by Stafford I Cohen July 26, 2011...With permission

20. David Kaplan interviewed by Stafford I Cohen February 11, 2011...With permission

21. Ibid

22. A Stone Freedberg MD interviewed by Stafford I Cohen March 08, 2006 and April 19, 2006. A Stone was Director of Research in the Department of Medicine. He helped Paul launch his career with grants, personnel, laboratory space and patient referrals. With permission

23. Zoll PM. The relation of tonal volume, intensity and pitch. Am J Psychol 1934; 46: 99-106

24. Zoll PM. The pluridimentionality of consciousness. Am J Psychol 1934; 46: 621-26

25. Zoll PM, Weiss S. Electrocardiographic changes in rats deficient in Vitamin B_1. Proc Soc Exp Biol Med 1936; 35: 259-62

26. Weiss S, Haynes FW, Zoll PM. Electrocardiographic manifestations and the cardiac effect of drugs in vitamin B_1 deficiency in rats. Am Heart J 1938; 15: 206-220

27. Ross Zoll interviewed by Stafford I Cohen February 09, 2009...With permission

28. Schlesinger MJ. An injection plus dissection study of coronary occlusions and anastomosis. Am Heart J 1938; 15: 528-68

29. Mary Zoll interviewed by Stafford I Cohen November 03, 2012...With permission

30. Nancy C Andreason MD, PhD. The Creating Brain. The Neuroscience of Genius. New York: Dana Press, 2005: 11-13

31. Arthur Linenthal MD interviewed by Kirk Jeffrey September 21, 1991. Arthur was one of Paul's long term collaborators and colleagues. With permission to reference the selected content from the NASPE/ HEART RHYTHM SOCIETY Rhythm in Time interviews

FOUR

1. Norman Morris. Ghetto Memories. Growing Up In Dorchester-Roxbury-Mattapan. self published, 2003

2. Ross Zoll interviewed by Stafford I Cohen February 29, 2009. With permission

3. Ibid

4. Lael Wertenbaker. To Mend the Heart. New York: Viking Press, 1980: 22

5. Ibid: 21

6. Ibid: 22

7. Alden Harken, personal communication August 17, 2009. With permission

8. Paul Axelrod interviewed by Stafford I Cohen October 01, 2009. With permission

9. Harken D, Zoll PM. Foreign bodies in and in relation to the thoracic blood vessels and heart III. Indications for the removal of intracardiac foreign bodies and the behavior of the heart during manipulation. Am Heart J 1946; 32: 1-19. In an interview, Dwight Harken cites 19 fragments in the heart chambers and 134 shell fragments in or about the great vessels. Dwight Harken interviewed by Gerald Rainer July 14, 2004. http://www.ctsnet.org/sections/residents/pioneer interviews/article-1.html

10. Gray Turner G. A bullet in the heart for twenty-three years. Surgery 1941; 9: 832-52

11. Decker HR. Foreign bodies in the heart and pericardium-should they be removed? J Thorac Surg 1939; 9: 62-9

12. Lael Wertenbaker. To Mend the Heart...1980: 43

13. Harken D, Zoll PM. Foreign bodies...Am Heart J 1946...Dwight Harken interviewed by Gerald Rainer...July 14, 2004

14. David Kaplan interviewed by Stafford I Cohen February 11, 2009. With permission

15. Zoll PM. Historical development of cardiac pacemakers. Prog Cardiovasc Dis. 1972; 14: 422

16. Associated Press. Cheney shooting victim suffers mild heart attack. Metro February 15, 2006: 1

17. Bryan Bender, Michael Kranish. Hunter shot by Cheney has a heart attack. The Boston Globe February 15, 2006: 1

18. Harken D, Zoll PM. Foreign bodies...Am Heart J 1946; 32: 1-19

19. Daniel Shugurensky, ed. History of Education: Selected Moments of the 20th Century. Chapter 1944 GI Bill of Rights. http//www.weir.ca/daniel_ shugurens/assignment1/1944gibill.html

20. Ibid

21. Tom Brokaw. The Greatest Generation. New York: Random House Trade Paperbacks, 1998: XXXVIII

22. Leona Norman Zarsky interviewed by Stafford I Cohen March 22, 2006. With permission

FIVE

1. Charles Lipson MD interviewed by Stafford I Cohen March 24, 2006. With permission

2. Lael Wertenbaker. To Mend the Heart. New York: The Viking Press, 1980: 22

3. Kyle Buckley. Dr. Paul M. Zoll: Pacemaker work saved thousands. PRN (Beth Israel Hospital) Spring 1993: 10

4. Schechter DC. Background of clinical cardiac electrostimulation III Electrical regulation of rapid cardiac dysrhythimas. NY State J Med 1972; 72: 281
To see an archival film of Claude Beck speaking to "The Choir of the Dead," go to www.hrsonline.org/News/ep-history/topics-in-death/index.cfm.Film title "Life and Death Relationship" 1958

5. Zoll PM. Historical development of cardiac pacing, MCVQ 1971; 7(4): 128

6. Condorelli L. Tentative de terapia in syndrome. Adams-Strokes. Ritmovenrivolare artificial mente mantenuto per due ore mediante stimulazioni mechanic. Minerva Med 1928; 8: 344-50.Translated by Francesca Delling MD. With permission

7. Schechter DC. Background of clinical cardiac...NY State J Med 1972; 72: 281

8. Harken DE, Ellis LB, Norman L. The surgical treatment of mitral stenosis II Progress in developing a controlled valvuloplastic technique. J Thorac Surg; 19: 1-15

9. Leona Norman Zarsky interviewed by Stafford I Cohen March 22, 2006. With permission

10. Zoll PM. A history of electrical cardiac stimulation. In Cardiac Pacing. Thalen HJTh, ed. Groinger, The Netherlands: Van Gorcum & Comp. B.V. Assen –The Netherlands, 1973: 6

11. Allen B Weisse MD. Heart To Heart. The Twentieth Century Battle Against Cardiac Disease. New Brunswick, New Jersey and London: Rutgers University Press, 2002: 160

12. Callaghan JC, Bigelow WG. An electrical artificial pacemaker for standstill of the heart. Thirty-Sixth Clinical Congress of the American College of Surgeons. Boston Massachusetts, October 1950. Philadelphia: WB Sanders Co,1951. Abstract: 265

13. Wilford G Bigelow. Cold Hearts. The Story Of Hypothermia And the Pacemaker In Heart Surgery. Toronto, Ontario: McClelland and Stewart Limited. The Canadian Publishers, 1984: 90

14. John A Hopps. Passing Pulses. The Pacemaker And Medical Engineering: A Canadian Story. Ottawa, Ontario: Publishing Plus Limited, 1955: 35

15. Allen B Weisse MD. Heart To Heart. The Twentieth Century Battle... New Brunswick, New Jersey and London: Rutgers University Press, 2002: 161

16. Zoll PM. Resuscitation of the heart in ventricular standstill by external electrical stimulation. N Engl J Med 1952; 249: 768-71

17. A. Stone Freedberg MD interviewed by Stafford I Cohen March 08, 2006. With permission

18. Ibid

19. Mr. A, the first closed-chest pacing success, can be viewed along with the Grass stimulator on the Heart Rhythm Society website. The subject of the film is Mr. A, who died at home six months after discharge from hospital. Dr. Zoll mentions the filming procedure in reference 23 below: page 164. For the film, go to www.hrsonline.org/News/ep-history/topics-in-death/index.cfm

20. Seymour Furman with Evelyn Furman interviewed by Victor Parsonnet April 11, 2001. With permission to reference the selected content from NASPE/HEART RHYTHM SOCIETY Rhythm in Time interviews

21. Aubrey Leatham: A real cardiologist pioneer from 20th Century – who has devoted his life to bedside cardiology and cardiac pacing. An interview by Dr. Ömer Göktekin. Anadolu Kardiol Derg, 2005; 5: 350

22. Aubrey Leatham. Correspondence to Stafford I Cohen July 05, 2011. With permission

23. Allen B Weisse MD. Heart To Heart. The Twentieth Century Battle...New Brunswick, New Jersey: Rutgers University Press, 2002: 165

24. K Patrick Ober. Mark Twain And Medicine. "Any mummery will cure." Columbia and London: University of Missouri Press, 2003: 261

25. Mr. A, the first closed-chest pacing success…www.hrsonline.org/News/ep-history/topics-in-death/index.cfm

26. Bigelow WG, Callaghan JC, Hopps JA. General hypothermia for experimental intracardiac surgery. Transactions of Seventieth Meeting of the American Surgical Association J.B. Lippincott Company 1950: 213. (See reference 34 below)

27. Weirich WL, Gott VL, Lillehei CW. The treatment of complete heart block by the combined use of a myocardial electrode and an artificial pacemaker. Surg Forum 1958; 8: 360-63

28. Glenn WWL, Mauro A, Longo E, Lavietes PH, MacKay FJ. Remote stimulation of the heart by radiofrequency transmission. Clinical application to a patient with Stokes-Adams syndrome. N Engl J Med 1959; 261: 948-51

29. Harken DE. Pacemakers, past-makers, and the paced: an informal history from A to Z (Aldini to Zoll). Biomed Instrum Technol 1991 Jul-Aug; 25: 319

30. Alan Belgard interviewed by Stafford I Cohen April 05, 2006. With permission

31. Alan Belgard interviewed by Stafford I Cohen February 06, 2007. With permission

32. Day HW. A cardiac resuscitation program. J-Lancet 1962; 82: 153-56

33. Alan Belgard interviewed by Stafford I Cohen April 05, 2006. With permission

34. Albert M Grass. The Electroencephalopathic Heritage. Grass Instrument Company, Quincy, MA 1984: 32.(see reference 26 above)

35. Paul Zoll interviewed by Kirk Jeffrey February 05, 1990. With permission to reference the selected content from the NASPE/HEART RHYTHM SOCIETY Rhythm in Time interviews.

36. Thomas S Kuhn. The Structure Of Scientific Revolutions. Chicago: The University of Chicago Press, 1996: Third Edition

SIX

1. Editorial. Electric stimulation in cardiac arrest. N Engl J Med 1952; 247: 781-82

2. The Bible. 2 Kings; chapter vs: 32-5

3. Schechter DC. Role of the humane societies in the history of resuscitation. Surg Gynecol Obstet 1969; 129: 811-15

4. Wendy Moore. The Knife Man. The Extraordinary Life and Times Of John Hunter, Father Of Modern Surgery. New York: Broadway Books, 2005: 189

5. David Charles Schechter. Electrical Cardiac Stimulation. Direct Electrostimulation Of Heart Without Thoracotomy. Minneapolis, MN: Medtronic Inc,1983: 91

6. Earl E Bakken. One Man's Full Life. Minneapolis, MN; Medtronic Inc, 1999: 92

7. Zoll PM. The intermediate history of cardiac pacing. In Harthorne JW, Thalen HJTh, eds. Boston Colloquium on Cardiac Pacing; The Hague-The Netherlands; Martinus Nijhoff Medical Division, 1976: 28

8. Milton Paul interviewed by Stafford I Cohen November 16, 2007. With permission

9. Zoll PM. The intermediate history of cardiac pacing...Boston Colloquium on Cardiac Pacing, 1976: 29

10. A Stone Freedberg interviewed by Stafford I Cohen March 08, 2006 and April 19, 2006. With permission

11. Leona Norman Zarsky interviewed by Stafford I Cohen March 22, 2006. With permission

12. Zoll PM. The intermediate history of cardiac pacing...Boston Colloquium on Cardiac Pacing, 1976: 29

13. Allen B Weisse MD. Heart To Heart. An Oral History. New Brunswick, New Jersey and London: Rutgers University Press, 2002: 176

14. The Theology for Everyman. Can a Dead Person Be Restored to Life? The Pilot February 12, 1955: 1

15. Moe GK. Oscillating course in arrhythmia research; a personal account. Int J Cardiol 1984; 5: 109-13

16. Eisenberg MS. Defibrillation: The spark of life. Scientific American 1998; June: 86-90

17. Allen B Weisse MD. Heart To Heart...New Brunswick, New Jersey and London; Rutgers University Press, 2002: 160

18. Beck CS, Pritchard WH, Feil HS. Ventricular fibrillation of long duration abolished by electrical shock. JAMA 1947; 135; 985-86

19. Beck CS, Leighniger DS. Death after a clean bill of health. JAMA 1960; 174: 133-35

20. Schechter DC, Background of clinical cardiac electrostimulation, III Electrical regulation of rapid cardiac dysrhythmias. NY State J of Med 1972; 72: 281

21. Allen B Weisse MD. Heart To Heart...New Brunswick, New Jersey and London: Rutgers University Press, 2002: 170

22. Zoll PM. Prevention and treatment of ventricular fibrillation and ventricular asystole. In Sudden Cardiac Death. Surawicz G, ed. New York and London: Grune & Stratton Inc, 1964: 151

23. Cardiac Resuscitation. Hurst JW, ed. Springfield IL: Charles C Thomas Publisher, 1960: 110.

24. Kouwenhoven KB, Jude JR, Knickerbocker GG. Closed-chest cardiac massage. JAMA 1960; 73: 94-7

25. Elam JO. Rediscovery of expired air methods for emergency ventilation. In Advances In Cardiopulmonary Resuscitation. Safer P, Elam JO, eds. New York: Springer-Verlag, 1977: chapter 39: 261-65

26. Marmorstein M. Contributions à létude des excitations électriques localisées sur le ceuer en rapport avec la topographic de linervation du coer chez le chien. Journal de Physiologic et de Patholgie General in Paris 1927; 25: 617

27. Wilford Bigelow and John Callaghan interviewed by Seymour Furman August 15, 1996. With permission to reference the selected content from the NASPE/HEART RHYTHM SOCIETY Rhythm in Time interviews

28. Callaghan JC. History. Early experiences in the development of an artificial electrical pacemaker for standstill of the heart. View from 1949. PACE 1980; 3: 618

29. Ibid

30. Callaghan JC, Bigelow WF. An electrical artificial pacemaker for standstill of the heart. Thirty-sixth Clinical Congress of the American College of Surgeons Boston Massachusetts October 1950. Philadelphia. London: WB Saunders Company, 1951; Abstract: 265

31. Wilford G Bigelow. Cold Hearts. The Story Of Hypothermia and the Pacemaker In Heart Surgery. Chapter four, The pacemaker: A cold heart spin-off. Toronto, Ontario: McLelland and Stewart. The Canadian Publisher, 1984: 106

32. Excerpts from Bigelow WG. Cold Hearts. The Story Of Hypothermia and the Pacemaker In Heart Surgery. Chapter four. PACE 1987; 10: 142-50

33. Zoll PM. Letter to the Editor. PACE 1987; 10: 1388

34. Bigelow WG. Letter to the Editor. PACE 1988; 11: 471

35. Äke Senning. Cardiac pacing in retrospect. Amer J Surg 1983; 145: 733-39

36. John A Hopps. Passing Pulses. The Pacemaker and Medical Engineering. A Canadian Story. Ottawa, Ontario; Publishing Plus Limited, 1995: 40

37. Ibid: 44

38. Wilford Bigelow interviewed by Seymour Furman August 14, 1996. With permission to reference the selected content from the NASPE/HEART RHYTHM SOCIETY Rhythm in Time interviews

39. Wilford Bigelow and John Callaghan interviewed by Seymour Furman August 15, 1996. With permission. Continuation of Dr. Furman's Rhythm in Time interviews (reference 38 above)

40. David KC Cooper. Open Heart. The Radical Surgeons Who Revolutionized Medicine. New York: Kaplan Publishing, 2010: 114

41. Ibid

42. John A Hopps. Passing Pulses... A Canadian Story...Publishing Plus Limited, 1955: 40

43. Allen B Weisse MD. Heart To Heart... New Brunswick, New Jersey and London: Rutgers University Press, 2010: 161

44. Hopps JA, Bigelow WG. Electrical treatment of cardiac arrest: A cardiac stimulator defibrillator. Surgery 1954; 36: 838

45. Alan Belgard interviewed by Stafford I Cohen April 14, 2006 and February 06, 2007, and correspondence dated April 11, 2008, June 11, 2011 and June 18, 2011. With permission

46. In the course of Wilford Bigelow being interviewed by Seymour Furman (reference #39), Furman was given a copy of the letter written by Zoll to Callaghan. The author (Stafford I Cohen) requested a copy of the letter from archivists at Toronto General Hospital and the Heart Rhythm Society who were unable to locate the letter within their collections

SEVEN

1. Cohen L, Conde CA. Ventricular arrhythmias during the hyperacute, acute and convalescent phases of myocardial infarction. In Acute Myocardial Infarction. Donoso E and Lipski I, eds. Current Cardiovascular Topics Vol. IV. New York, Stratton International Medical Book Corp, 1978: 112-68

2. Engineering Staff of Fentosim Clinical Inc. History of physiological monitors. Fifty years of physiological monitors. http://fentosimclinical,com/History%20of%20Physiologic%20Monitors.

3. Zoll PM, Linenthal AJ, Norman LR, Paul MH, Gibson W. External electrical stimulation of the heart in cardiac arrest. Arch Int Med 1955; 96: 647

4. Furman S. Forward to The Making Of The Pacemaker. Greatbatch W. Amherst, NY: Promethius Books, 2000: 13

5. Zoll PM. Resuscitation of the heart in ventricular standstill by external electric stimulation. N Engl J Med 1952; 247: 768-81

6. Zoll PM, Linenthal AJ, Norman LR, Belgard AH. Treatment of Stokes-Adams disease by external electric stimulation of the heart. Circulation 1954; 9: 482-93

7. Leatham A, Cook P, Davies JG. External electric stimulator for treatment of ventricular standstill. Lancet 1956; 2: 1185-89

8. Ibid

9. Aubrey Leatham. Correspondence to Stafford I Cohen February 05, 2007. With permission

10. Aubrey Leatham interviewed by Seymour Furman June 23, 1996. With permission to reference the selected content from the NASPE/HEART RHYTHM SOCIETY Rhythm in Time interviews

11. Aubrey Leatham. Draft of Geoffrey Davies' Obituary October 18, 2008. With permission

12. Aubrey Leatham. Correspondence to Stafford I Cohen...With permission

13. Furman S, Schwedel JB. An intracardiac pacemaker for Stokes-Adams seizures. N Engl J Med 1959; 261: 943-48

14. Leatham A, Rickards A, Gold R. Cardiac Pacing. In British Cardiology in the 20th Century. Silverman ME, Fleming PR, Hollman A, Julian DG, Krikler DM, eds. London: Springer-Verlag, 2000: 214
    The terms Automatic Pacing, Ventricular Inhibited Pacing and Demand Pacing are not interchangeable. Although each type of pacing starts when there is absence of cardiac activity for a specified interval, each type of pacing terminates under different circumstances. Automatic Pacing by Electrodyne was manually terminated. Leatham and Davies' advanced pacer was ventricular inhibited, which meant that the device would self-terminate pacing when the heart resumed beating at an average rate that was at an adequate level for a specified period of time. Although Leatham termed his advanced pacer a Demand Pacemaker, it was judged not to fulfill that strict definition in a patent infringement law-suit, which ruled that Demand Pacing is governed by a

pacemaker's response to the rate determined by the interval between two sequential heart beats, rather than by the average rate of a number of beats

15. More Than 20 Here Owe Lives to Heart Starter. Boston Daily Globe February 15, 1955, with an image of Mrs. Colin McKenzie. Another image was wired by the Associated Press and appeared in The Kerrville Texas Times February 18, 1955 and The New York Daily News February 17, 1955

16. Correspondence dated October 24, 1955 relating to a purchase order dated August 08, 1955. Courtesy of Alan Belgard. With permission

17. New England Hospital Officials Gather. Boston Globe March 26,1956. An image of the PM-65 is included

18. Pacemakers Presented By the Rhode Island Heart Association and Miriam Hospital. Providence Journal July 29, 1956. The pacemakers are Electrodyne model PM-65s

19. Purchase order dated July 10, 1956. Courtesy of Alan Belgard. With permission

20. Twenty Ninth Scientific Sessions of the American Heart Association. October 26-29, 1956. Technical exhibits. Circulation 1956; 14: 682

21. Zoll PM...External stimulation of the heart in cardiac arrest. Arch Int Med 1955; 96: 647

22. Zoll PM, Linenthal AJ, Norman LR, Paul MH, Gibson W. Treatment of unexpected cardiac arrest by external electric stimulation of the heart. N Engl J Med 1956; 254: 541-46

23. Zoll PM, Linenthal AJ, Zarsky LRN. Ventricular fibrillation. Treatment and prevention by external currents. N Engl J Med 1960; 262: 105-112

24. Zoll PM. Historical development of cardiac pacemakers. Prog Cardiovasc Dis 1972; 14: 424

25. Zoll PM. A history of electric cardiac stimulation. In Cardiac Pacing. Thalin HJTh, ed. Groinger, The Netherlands: Van Gorcum & Comp. B.V., Assen-The Netherlands, 1973: 8

26. Zoll PM. Development of electric control of cardiac rhythm. JAMA 1973; 226: 884

27. Personal observation. Stafford I Cohen

28. Mark Twain. A Connecticut Yankee In King Arthur's Court. Chapter XXVI. The first newspaper

29. Personal observation. Stafford I Cohen

30. Heart Rhythm Society. Electricity and the Heart. Tony's Cardiac Pacemaker. http://hrs.nusura.com/1957ScienceReport.php

31. The film of Tony's Cardiac Pacemaker was salvaged from Dr. Leona Norman Zarsky's home attic and given to the Heart Rhythm Society to archive by Stafford I Cohen

32. Liz Kowalczyk. Patient alarms often unheard, unheeded. Part One. Boston Sunday Globe February 13, 2011: A1,A14-15. Liz Kowalczk. No easy solutions for alarm fatigue. Hospitals examine overuse. Part Two. The Boston Globe February 14, 2011: A1,A8

33. Liz Kowalczyk. "Alarm fatigue" a factor in second death. The Boston Globe September 21, 2011: A1,A7

34. Liz Kowalczyk. Hospitals warned of alarm fatigue. The Boston Globe April 9, 2013: B1,B13

EIGHT

1. Zoll PM, Linenthal AJ. External and internal electric cardiac pacemakers. Circulation 1963; 28: 455-56

2. Walter Issacson. No mere genius. Special Einstein Issue Discover 2004; 25: 12-14

3. Alan Belgard interviewed by Stafford I Cohen April 04, 2006. With permission

4. Alan Belgard's description is derived from interviews and correspondence as follows: Alan Belgard interviewed by Stafford I Cohen April 04, 2006 and February 06, 2007. With permission. Alan Belgard correspondence to Stafford I Cohen June 08, 2011. With permission

5. Furman S, Schwedel JB. An intracardiac pacemaker for Stokes-Adams seizures. N Engl J Med 1959; 261: 943-48

6. David Quirk. His heart plugged in. Currently he's swell. Daily News November 27, 1958

NINE

1. Seymour Furman with Evelyn Furman interviewed by Victor Parsonett April 11, 2001. With permission to reference the selected content from the NASPE/HEART RHYTHM SOCIETY Rhythm in Times interviews

2. Furman S, Robinson G. The use of an intracardiac pacemaker in the correction of total heart block. Surg Forum 1959; Vol IX: 245-48

3. Furman S, Schwedel JB. An intracardiac pacemaker for Stokes-Adams seizures. N Engl J Med 1959; 261: 943-48

4. Furman S. Recollections of the beginnings of transvenous pacing. PACE 1994; 17: 1697-1705

5a-5f. Earl E Bakken. One Man's Full Life. Minneapolis, MN: Medtronics Inc, 1999: 49. (b) C Walton Lillehei's biographer G Wayne Miller writes that the tragic baby death during the 1957 Halloween power outage is "rumor". King of Hearts. New York: Random House. Times Book Division, 2000: 105. (c) G Wayne Miller repeats that the death was only rumor. Into the heart-a medical odyssey. Unexpected outcomes. Cross-Circulation. http://www.projo.com/specials/heart/8b.htm (d) Lillehei remembers the blackout, but not the death. C. Walton Lillehei interviewed by Kirk Jeffrey July 25, 1990. With permission to reference the selected content from the NASPE/HEART RHYTHM SOCIETY Rhythm in Times interviews. (e) Earl Bakken has clear recall of Lillehei's distress following the child's death. Janet Moore. Pacemaker keeps the beat going on. Star Tribune December 08, 2007 (f) Vincent Gott, a Lillehei trainee, refers to the October 31, 1957 blackout without reference to a patient death on the premise that the hospital had alternative electric power. Gott VL. Critical role of physiologist John A Johnson in the origins of Minnesota's billion dollar pacemaker industry. Ann Thorac Surg 2007; 83: 349-53. Earl Bakken, however, notes that the backup generator only powered selected areas, but not patient rooms

6. Earl E Bakken. One Man's Full Life...Medtronics Inc, 1999: 50

7. Furman S. Recollections of the beginnings... PACE 1994; 17: 1697-705

8a-8c. Robert C. Toth. Has electric wire in heart 96 days. New York Herald Tribune November 27, 1958. (b) David Quirk. His heart plugged in. Currently he's swell. Daily News November 27, 1958. (c) Pacemaker out; Cardiac patient leaves hospital. Scope Weekly December 08, 1958

9. Zoll PM. Resuscitation of the heart in ventricular standstill by external electrical stimulation. N Engl J Med 1952; 247: 768-71

10. Seymour Furman with Evelyn Furman interviewed by Victor Parsonett April 11, 2001. With permission

11. Furman S. Recollections of the beginnings...PACE 1994; 17: 1697-705

12. Furman S, Schwedel JB. An intracardiac pacemaker... N Engl J Med 1959; 261: 943-48

13. Marcel Zimetbaum MD. Personal communication, February 18, 2008. With permission

TEN

1. Zoll PM. Resuscitation of the heart in ventricular standstill by external electrical stimulation. N Engl J Med 1952; 247: 761-71

2. Zoll PM, Linenthal AJ, Gibson W, Paul MH, Norman LR. Termination of ventricular fibrillation in man by externally applied countershock. N Engl J Med 1956; 254: 727-32

3. Abeldgaard PC. Tentamina electrica in animalibus institute. Societatis Medicae Havniensis Collectanae 1775; 2: 157-61

4. Chamberlain D. Never quite there: a tale of resuscitation medicine. In Resuscitation Greats. Baskett PJF and Baskett TF, eds. Redland, Bristol: Clinical Press Ltd, 2007: 356

5. Driscol TE, Ratnoff OD, Nygaard OF. The remarkable Dr. Abildgaard [sic] and countershock. The bicentennial of his electrical experiments on animals. Ann Int Med 1975; 83: 878-82

6. MacWilliam JA. Fibrillar contraction of the heart. J Physiol 1887; 8: 296-310

7. McWilliam JA. Cardiac failure and sudden death. Br Med J 1889; 1: 6-8

8. Prevost JL, Battelli F. La mort par les courants electriques alternatives a houte tension. Journal de Physiologie et de Pathologie General 1899; 1: 399-412 and 11: 427-42

9. Hooker DR, Kouwenhoven WB, Langworthy OR. The effect of alternating electric currents on the heart. Am J Physiol 1933; 103: 444-54

10a. Carl Wiggers. Reminiscences and Adventures in Circulation Research. New York and London: Grune and Stratton, 1958: 282

10b. Paul Zoll interviewed by Kirk Jeffrey September 19, 1991. With permission

10c. Allen B Weisse MD, Heart to Heart. an oral history. Interview with Paul M Zoll. New Brunswick, New Jersey and London: Rutgers University Press, 2002: 169-70

11. Zoll PM. The intermediate history of cardiac pacing. In Boston Colloquium on Cardiac Pacing. Harthorne JW and Thalen HJTh, eds. The Hague-The Netherlands: The Martinus Nijoff Medical Division,1977: 29

12. Gurvich NL, Yuniev GS. Restoration of regular rhythm in the mammalian fibrillating heart. Am Rev Soviet Med 1946; 3: 236-39

13. Gurvich NL, Yuniev GS. Restoration of heart rhythm during fibrillation by a condenser discharge. Am Rev Soviet Med 1947; 4: 253-56

14. Leona Norman Zarsky interviewed by Stafford I Cohen March 22, 2006. With permission

15. Zoll PM, Linenthal AJ...Termination of ventricular...N Engl J Med 1956; 254: 727-32

16. Victor Gurewich interviewed by Stafford I Cohen October 23, 2008. With permission

17. Zoll PM, Linenthal AJ...Termination of ventricular...N Engl J Med 1956; 254: 727-32

18a. Zoll PM. Countershock and pacemaking in cardiac arrhythmias. Hosp Pract 1975; 10: 125-32

18b. Zoll PM. Cardiac stimulation and countershock. Early experiences. In 3rd Einhoven Meeting in Past and Present Cardiology. Theme: Arrhythmias. Artzenius AC, Dunning AJ, Snellen HA, eds. Leiden, Netherlands: Spruyt, Van Mantgem & DeDoes, 1984: 114-120

19. Documents on file with Stafford I Cohen

20. Guyton AC, Satterfield J. Factors concerned in electrical defibrillation of the heart, particularly through the unopened chest. Am J Physiol 1951; 167: 81-87

21a. Kouwenhoven WB, Milnor WR, Knickerbocker BS, Chestnut WR. Closed chest defibrillation of the heart. Surgery 1957; 42: 550-61. The first success is described on pages 559-60

21b. Kouwenhoven WB. The development of the defibrillator. Ann Int Med 1969; 71: 449-58. The date of their first success was March 28 1957

22. Knickerbocker G. Contributions of William B Kouwenhoven–Reminiscences. In 1975 Wolf Creek Conference on Advances in Cardiopulmonary Resuscitation. Safer P, Elam J, eds. New York: Springer-Verlag, 1977: 255-258

23. Kouwenhoven WB, Knickerbocker GG, Becker EM. Portable defibrillator. IEEE Trans Power Apparatus & Systems 1963; No 6: 1089-93

24. Kouwenhoven WB. The development of the defibrillator. Ann Int Med 1969; 71: 449-57

25. James Jude and Guy Knickerbocker interviewed by Stafford I Cohen December 09, 2010. With permission

26. Acosta P, Varon J, Sternbach GL, Baskett P. Kouwenhoven, Jude and Knickerbocker. The introduction of defibrillation and external chest compression into modern resuscitation. In Resucitation Greats. Baskett PJF, Baskett TF, eds. Redlands, Bristol, UK: Clinical Press Ltd 2007: 262-66

27. Maass F. Die method der wiederbelenbung bei herztod nach chloroformeinathmung. Berliner Klinische Wochenschrift 1892; 12: 265-8. Referenced in Fugi M, Pelinka LE, Mauritz W, Koenig F, Maass F. Resuscitation Greats. Baskett PGF, Baskett TF, eds. Redland, Bristol UK: Clinical Press Ltd, 2007: 151-54

28. Jude JR. Personal reminiscences of the origin and history of cardiopulmonary resuscitation (CPR). Am J Cardiol 2003; 8: 956-63

29. Kouwenhoven WB, Jude JR, Knickerbocker GG. Closed-chest cardiac massage. JAMA 1960; 173: 1064-67

30. Cakulev I, Efimov IR, Waldo AL. Cardioversion: past, present and future. Circulation 2009; 120: 1623-32

31. Gurvich NL...Restoration of regular rhythm... Am Rev Soviet Med 1946; 3: 326-39

32. Gurvich NL...Restoration of heart rhythm... Am Rev Soviet Med 1947; 4: 253-56

33. Cakulev I, Efimov IR, Waldo AL. Cardioversion: past, present and future. Circulation 2009...which references instructions on the application of methods to resuscitate life functions in the terminally ill. In USSR Ministry of Health, ed: Medgiz; 1959

34. Ibid: 1625

35. James Jude and Guy Knickerbocker interviewed ...December 09, 2010

36. Negovsky VA. Fifty years of the Institute of General Reanimatology of the USSR Academy of Medical Sciences. Crit Care Med 1988; 16: 288

37. Bernard Lown. Prescription for Survival. San Francisco: Berrett-Koehler Publishers Inc, 2008: 32-46

38. Cukulev I, Effimov JR...Cardioversion: past, present...Circulation 2009; 120: 1623-32

39. Personal experience. Stafford I Cohen

40. Albert Morris interviewed by Stafford I Cohen September 09, 1998. With permission

ELEVEN

1. Albert Morris. Correspondence to Stafford I Cohen February 21, 2008. With permission

2. Albert Morris. Correspondence to Stafford I Cohen March 08, 2008. With permission

3. Letter from Albert Morris to Mickey Eisenberg September 09, 1998. With permission of Albert Morris

4. Albert Morris interviewed by Stafford I Cohen March 05, 2009. With permission

5. Memorandum from Albert Morris to business associates dated February 24, 1998 with attachment titled Prospectus On Morris Defibrillator Company, Circa 1951-1952. With permission

6. Albert Morris. Correspondence...March 08, 2008. With permission

7. Notable Figures in EP History. http://www.hrsonline.org/ep-history/notable_figures/bios/claude_beck

8. For an image of the Beck-Rand defibrillator, http://www.thebakken.org/artifacts/beck-defibrillator.htm

9. Albert Morris interviewed by Stafford I Cohen May 23, 2008. With permission

10. Albert Morris. Sales training tape for salesmen regarding defibrillators, pacemakers and resuscitation. April 01, 1954. With permission

11. Albert Morris interviewed...May 23, 2008. With permission

12. Acierno LJ, Worrel T. George Ralph Mines: Victim of self experimentation? Clin Cardiol 2001; 224: 571-72

13. Lüdernitz B, ed. History. George Ralph Mines (1886-1914). J Interv Card Electrophysiol 2005; 12: 163-64

14. Albert Morris interviewed...May 23, 2008. With permission

15. Tom Corbin. Corrspondence to Stafford I Cohen July 01, 2009. With permission

16. Kouwenhoven WB. The development of the defibrillator. Ann Int Med 1969; 71: 449-58

17. Earl E Bakken. One Man's Full Life. Minneapolis, MN: Medtronics Inc, 1999: 43

18. Albert Morris interviewed...March 05, 2009. With permission

19. Zoll PM, Linenthal AJ, Norman LR, Belgard AH. Treatment of Stokes-Adams disease by external electric stimulation of the heart. Circulation 1954; 9; 482

20. Alan Belgard. Correspondence to Stafford I Cohen March 02, 2013. With permission

21. Albert Morris interviewed...March 05, 2009. With permission

22. Albert Morris interviewed...May 23, 2008. With permission

23. Paul Zoll interviewed by Kirk Jeffrey February 05, 1990. With permission

24. Memorandum from Albert Morris...February 24, 1998. Prospectus On Morris Defibrillator Company, Circa 1951-1952. With permission

25. Albert Morris interviewed...May 23, 2008. With permission

26. ZMI Corporation vs. Physio-Control Corporation 1988. United States District Court. Western District of Washington, at Seattle. NO. C86-726(C)WD. P. 839

27. Correspondence regarding a testimonial praising the successful performance of a Morris Clinical Pacemaker March 02, 1955 and July 05, 1955

28. Zoll PM, Linenthal AJ, Norman LR, Paul MH, Gibson W. External electrical stimulation of the heart in cardiac arrest. Arch Int Med 1955; 96: 639-53

29. Albert Morris. Correspondence to Stafford I Cohen June 14, 2008. With permission

30. Attempts by the author, Stafford I Cohen, to receive information through The Freedom of Information Act about the purchase and presence of cardiac defibrillators at the Aero Medical Laboratory at Wright-Patterson Air Base met with failure

31. Albert Morris interviewed... May 23, 2008. With permission

32. Tom Corbin. Harthrob. Kahului, Hawaii: QRS INC. Produced by Jungle Press, 1944: 71

33. Neville PC, Bondurant S, Leverett SD. Human tolerance to prolonged forward and backward acceleration. J Aviat Med 1959; 30: 1-21

34. Urshel CW, Hood WB Jr. Cardiovascular effect of rotation on Z axis. Aerospace Medical Research Labs Wright- Patterson AFB Ohio 1966. Abstract. Accession Number AD0634080

35. Kouwenhoven WB, Ing DR, Milnor WR, Knickerbocker GG, Chestnut WR. Closed chest defibrillation of the heart. Surgery 1957; 42: 550-56

36. Kouwenhoven WB. The development...Ann Int Med 1969; 71: 449-58

37. Curriculum vitae. Prepared by Albert Morris for Tom Morrin, Stanford Research Institute. January 26, 1962. With permission

TWELVE

1. Ross Zoll PhD MD. 50th Anniversary of defibrillation: Paul M Zoll MD and the beginning of Zoll Medical Corporation. EP Lab Digest 2006; 6: 14-16. Ross is Paul and Janet's son

2. A Stone Freedberg interviewed by Stafford I Cohen March 08, 2006. With permission

3. Personal observation by Stafford I Cohen

4. David Lewis MD. Correspondence to Stafford I Cohen April 02, 2009. David trained at Beth Israel Hospital and later joined the medical staff as a sub-specialist. With permission

5. Elliot Mahler interviewed by Stafford I Cohen September 29, 2007. Elliot is Paul's second cousin. With permission

6. Abelmann WH, Axelrod P, Cohen SI. Faculty of Medicine Memorial Minute. Harvard University Gazette; April 19, 2001: 12

7. Mary Zoll PhD interviewed by Stafford I Cohen July 26, 2011. Mary is Paul and Janet's daughter. With permission

8. Ibid

9. David Kaplan interviewed by Stafford I Cohen February 11, 2008. David is Paul's first cousin. With permission

10. Mary Zoll...interviewed by Stafford I Cohen July26, 2011. With permission

11. Violet Linenthal interviewed by Stafford I Cohen November 20, 2008. Violet is the wife of Arthur Linenthal MD. With permission

12. Ross Zoll PhD MD interviewed by Stafford I Cohen February 09, 2009. With permission

13. A Stone Freedberg...interviewed by Stafford I Cohen March 08, 2006. With permission

14. Mahler EJ. Memorial Service for Paul Maurice Zoll MD. Beth Israel Hospital February 23, 1999. Courtesy of the Ruth and David Freiman Archives at Beth Israel Deaconess Medical Center. With permission

15. Elliot Mahler interviewed by Stafford I Cohen September 29, 2007...With permission

16. Mahler EJ. Memorial Service... Beth Israel Hospital, February 23, 1999. Courtesy of the Ruth and David Freiman Archives... With permission

17. Freedberg AS. In Memoriam. Harvard Med Alumni Bull 1999; 72: 56-7

18. Mary Zoll interviewed by Stafford I Cohen July 26, 2011. With permission

19. Ibid

20. Ibid

21. Elsie Zoll interviewed by Stafford I Cohen March 22, 2006. Elsie is Paul Zoll's sister-in-law, Herbert's wife. With permission

22. Letter on file with Stafford I Cohen

23. Frederica Sigel interviewed by Stafford I Cohen February 08, 2008. Fredrica is a former neighbor and friend of Paul and Janet Zoll. With permission

24. Elliot Mahler…interviewed by Stafford I Cohen September 29, 2007. With permission

25. Mary MacIntyre. Paul Zoll's secretary. Correspondence to Stafford I Cohen September 14, 2011. With permission

26. Paul Zoll MD, having none of these "unhealthy habits," lived to age 87

27. Freedberg AS…In Memoriam…Med Alumni Bull 1999; 72: 56-7

28. Mary MacIntyre…Correspondence…With permission

29. Daphne Glassman. Next door neighbor of Paul and Janet Zoll. Correspondence to Stafford I Cohen, January 19, 2008. With permission

30. Ross Zoll…interviewed by Stafford I Cohen February 29, 2009. With permission

31. Sylvia Summers. Family member of a Paul Zoll patient. Correspondence to Stafford I Cohen, November 25, 2007. With permission

32. Fay Berzon RN. Nurse at Beth Israel Hospital and patient of Paul Zoll. Correspondence to Stafford I Cohen, January 05, 2008. With permission

33. Letters on file with Stafford I Cohen

34. Letters on file with Stafford I Cohen

35. Alan Belgard interviewed by Stafford I Cohen April 05, 2006. Alan is Paul's longstanding engineer and collaborator. With permission

36. Ross Zoll interviewed by Stafford I Cohen February 09, 2009. With permission

37. Leona Norman Zarsky MD interviewed by Stafford I Cohen March 22, 2006. Leona was a colleague, co-worker and co-author with Paul Zoll. With permission

38. Ibid

THIRTEEN

1. Stokes-Adams attacks are defined as fainting or near fainting spells from transient, sustained, or permanent failure of electrical transmission within the heart's conduction system that result in an inadequate heart rate to circulate blood to the brain

2. Arne & Else Marie Larsson interviewed by Seymour Furman June 29, 1999. With permission to reference the selected content from NASPE/HEART RHYTHM SOCIETY Rhythm in Time interviews
•Elmqvist R, Senning Ä. An implantable pacemaker for the heart. In Medical Electronics. Proceedings of the Second International Conference on Medical Electronics. Paris 24-27 June 1959. C.N. Smyth, ed. London: Iliffe & Sons Ltd., 1960: 253-54 (abstract)

3. Brunckhorst C, Candinas R, Furman S. Biography of Äke Senning. Heart Rhythm Society. http://www.hrsonline.org/News/ep-history/notable-figures/akesenning.cfm. This web site has been discontinued. Hard copy is on file with author

4. Electric pulses set the heart's pace. Siemens Review 1984; 51(2): 5-8

5. Senning Ä. Cardiac pacing in retrospect. Amer J Surg 1983; 145: 733-39

6. Siddons AHM, Humphries O'N. Complete heart block with Stokes-Adams attacks treated by indwelling pacemakers. Proc R Soc Med 1961; 54: 237-38

7. Paul Zoll interviewed by Kirk Jeffrey February 5, 1990. With permission to reference the selected content from NASPE/HEART RHYTHM SOCIETY Rhythm in Time interviews •Allen B Weisse MD. Heart to Heart. New Brunswick, New Jersey: Rutgers University Press, 2002: 168

8. David Charles Schechter. Exploring the Origins of Electrical Cardiac Stimulation. Chapter 9, Modern era of artificial cardiac pacemakers. Minneapolis, MN: Medtronic Inc, 1983: 114

9. Alan Belgard interviewed by Seymour Furman and S. Serge Barold August 18, 2001. With permission to reference the selected content from NASPE/HEART RHYTHM SOCIETY Rhythm in Time interviews

10. Harken D. Pacemakers, past-makers, and the paced: An informal history from A to Z (Aldino to Zoll). Biomed Instrum Technol 1991 Jul-Aug; 25(4): 319

11. Zoll PM, Frank HA, Zarsky LRN, Linenthal AJ, Belgard AH. Long-term electrical stimulation of the heart for Stokes-Adams disease. Ann Surg 1961; 154: 330-46

12. Merrill Cohen PhD. Correspondence to Stafford I Cohen December 18, 2009. With permission

13. Hunter SW, Roth NA, Bernardez D, Noble JL. A bipolar myocardial electrode for complete heart block. J Lancet 1959; 79: 506-08

14. Wilson Greatbatch. The Making of the Pacemaker. Amhurst, New York: Prometheus Books, 2000: 32

15. Chardack WM, Gage AA, Greatbatch W. A Transistorized self-contained implantable pacemaker for the long-term correction of complete heart block. Surgery 1960; 48: 643-45. Chardack and Greatbatch abandoned research on their own lead in favor of the Hunter-Roth design. Years later William Chardack developed a revolutionary concept for epicardial and endocardial leads based on a coiled spring design that was capable of more flexes with less breakage–thereby significantly extending functional lead longevity

16. Steven M Spencer. Making a heartbeat behave. The Saturday Evening Post March 4, 1961: 13-15,48,50

17. Kirk Jeffrey. Machines In Our Hearts. Baltimore, Maryland: Johns Hopkins University Press, 2001: 88,103

18. Heart Rhythm Foundation. Hrsonline. This public web site was discontinued. A segment of an Interview of William Glenn by Seymour Furman mentioned that WT was William Tobbler

19. Heart Rhythm Society. Electricity and the heart. Tony's cardiac pacemaker. http://hrs.nusura.com/1957ScienceReport.php

20. Glenn WWL, Mauro A, Longo E, Lavietes PH, MacKay FJ. Remote stimulation of the heart by radiofrequency transmission. Clinical application to a patient with Stokes-Adams Syndrome. N Engl J Med 1959; 261: 948-51

21. Mauro A. Technique for in-situ stimulation. Yale Biophys Bull 1948; 1: 2

22. Verseano M, Webb Jr RE, Kelly M. Radio control of ventricular contraction in experimental heart block. Science 1959; 128: 1003-04 (abstract)

23. William Glenn Interviewed by Seymour Furman May 04, 2001. With permission to reference the selected content from the NASPE/HEART RHYTHM SOCIETY Rhythm in Time interviews

24. Ibid

25. Alexander Mauro might have been aware of the October 31, 1957 Twin City three-hour blackout that claimed the life of one of Walton Lillehei's blue babies

26. Eisenberg L, Mauro A, Glenn WWL. Transistorized pacemaker for remote stimulation of the heart by radiofrequency transmission. Ire Trans Biomed Electron 1961; BME-8: 253

27. Sidney Levitsky interviewed by Stafford I Cohen March 19, 2008. With permission. Dr. Levitsky trained with Dr. William Glenn in cardiac surgery and spent a year as a Research Fellow in 1961 modifying the transistorized radiofrequency pacemaker. He visited the pacemaker patients at their homes and treated them during hospital clinic visits. Levitsky helped invent an auxiliary battery pack that permitted transmitter-battery replacement without interruption of pacing. Replacing transmitter batteries was recommended each three to four days

28. Levitsky S, Glenn WWL, Mauro A, Eisenberg L, Smith PW. Long-term stimulation of the heart with radiofrequency transmission. Surgery 1962; 52: 64-75

29. Windman WD, Glenn WWL, Eisenberg L, Mauro A. Radiofrequency cardiac pacemaker. Ann NY Acad Sci 1964; 111: 992-1006

30. Sidney Levitsky interviewed ... March 29, 2008. With permission

31. Zoll PM. Cardiac resuscitation and the internist. In Cardiac Resuscitation. Hurst JW, ed. Springfield, Illinois Charles C. Thomas, 1960: 46

32. Gene Lorick. "Built In" electronic device would spur faltering heart. Boston Traveler December 3, 1959: B53

33. Radio heart pacemaker envisioned by 2 scientists. The Stars and Stripes November 9, 1960: 5. The two scientists are Paul Zoll and Arthur Linenthal

34. Zoll PM, Linenthal AJ, Zarsky LN. Ventricular fibrillation. Treatment and prevention by external electric currents. N Engl J Med 1960; 262: 105-12

35. Zoll PM, Frank HA, Zarsky LRN,... Long-term electrical...Ann Surg 1961; 154: 333

36. Furman S, Young D, Cardiac pacing in children and adolescents. Amer J Cardiol 1977; 39: 550-58

37. Paul Zoll. During panel discussion IV. Andrew G. Morrow, Chairman. Ann NY Acad Sci 1964; 111: 1105

38. Zoll PM, Frank HA, Zarsky LRN,... Long-term electrical...Ann Surg 1961; 154: 335

39. Beryl Chapman RN interviewed by Stafford I Cohen December 13, 2009. With permission. Nurse Chapman witnessed Howard Frank performing the second stage of Michael Seiffer's operation. She recalled that the prototype pacemaker resembled a pack of Lucky Strike cigarettes, which confirms Alan Belgard's story of the evolving Electrodyne implantable pacemaker. She also recalled participating in the ritual of boiling the leads with their then gold needles in Ivory Flakes and preparing the pacemakers for implantation

40. Quote attributed to Antarctic explorer Robert Scott upon discovering that his Norwegian rival had reached the South Pole. In Caroline Alexander. The man who took the prize. National Geographic September 2011: 135.

41. Noah Gordon. Electronic device inserted in chest keeps heart going. Boston Herald September 15, 1960: 18A

42. Howard Frank MD interviewed by Kirk Jeffrey October 16, 1996. With permission

43. Zoll PM, Frank HA, Zarsky LRN...Long-term electrical...Ann Surg 1961; 154: 330-46

44. Noah Gordon. Electronic device...Boston Herald September 15, 1960: 18A

45. Gerald Rosenblatt MD. Correspondence to Stafford I Cohen July 11, 2004. With permission. Dr. Rosenblatt, a medical resident trainee in 1960, was an observer during Dr. Seiffer's operation

46. Leona Zarsky MD. Paul Zoll Memorial Service. Beth Israel Hospital. February 23, 1999. With permission

47. Zoll PM, Frank HA, Zarsky LRN... Long term electrical...Ann Surg 1961; 154: 330-46

48. Noah Gordon. Electronic device...Boston Herald September 15, 1960: 18A

49. Charles Lipson MD interviewed by Stafford I Cohen March 24, 2006. With permission. Dr. Lipson was a surgical trainee at Beth Israel Hospital in 1960

50. Zoll PM, Frank HA, Zarsky LRN...Long-term electrical...Ann Surg 1961; 154: 330-46

51. Kantrowitz A, Cohen R, Raillard H, Schmidt J. Experimental and clinical experience with a new implantable cardiac pacemaker. Circulation 1961; 24: 967 (abstract)

52. Donald McRae. Every Second Counts. The Race To Transplant the First Human Heart. New York: G. P. Putnam's Sons, 2006: 96-99

53. Ibid

54. Kantrowitz A. The treatment of Stokes-Adams Syndrome in heart block. Prog Cardiovasc Dis 1964; 6: 490-506. There are inconsistencies regarding patient Rose Cohen as described in medical reports by Adrian Kantrowitz and her characterization by biographer Donald McRae, who might have erred in writing that her age was in the twenties and that she was a full implant recipient of Kantrowitz's primitive pacemaker

55. Harken D. Pacemakers, past-makers, and the paced: ... Biomed Instrum Technol 1991 Jul-Aug; 25(4): 305

56. Zoll PM. The intermediate history of cardiac pacing. In: Harthorn JW, Thalen HJTh, eds. Boston Colloquium on Cardiac Pacing. The Hague-The Netherlands: Martinus Nijhoffs Medical Division, 1977: 32

FOURTEEN

1. Zoll PM. Resuscitation of the heart in ventricular standstill by external electrical stimulation. N Engl J Med 1952; 247: 768-71

2. Robert Cooke. Dr. Folkman's War. New York: Random House, 2001: 23

3. Folkman, JM, Watkins E. An artificial conduction system for the management of experimental complete heart block. Surg Forum 1958; 8: 331-34

4. The first atrial sensed-ventricular paced device was manufactured for patients by the Cordis Company in 1962, six years after Folkman and Watkin's publication. Nathan DA, Samet P, Center S, Chang YW. Long-term correction of complete heart block. Prog Cardiovasc Dis 1964; 6: 538-65

5. Robert Cook. Dr. Folkman's War...Random House: 37

6. Gott VL. Critical role of physiologist John A Johnson in the origins of Minnesota's billion dollar pacemaker industry. Ann Thorac Surg 2007; 83: 349-53

7. Folkman JM, Watkins E. An artificial conduction system...Surg Forum 1958; 8: 331-34

8. Weirich WL, Gott VL, Lillehei WC. The treatment of complete heart block by the combined use of a myocardial electrode and an artificial pacemaker. Surg Forum 1958; 8: 360-63

9. Zoll PM, Frank HA, Zarsky LRN, Linenthal AJ, Belgard AH. Long-term electrical stimulation of the heart for Stokes-Adams disease. Ann Surg 1961; 154: 338

10. Sells furniture, car to pay part of boy's bill; not complaining. The Daily Courier (Connellsville, PA) November 11, 1961: 9

11. Noah Gordon. "Best Thanksgiving ever" for boy 8, with battery-operated heart. Boston Herald November 24, 1960: 16

12. Ronald Meyer. Article appeared in an unknown Italian language newspaper. Courtesy of Alan Belgard. With permission. Translated by Francesca Delling MD. With permission

13. Noah Gordon. "Best Thanksgiving ever" ...Boston Herald November 24, 1960: 16

14. Chardack WM, Gage AA, Greatbatch W. Correction of complete heart block by a self-contained and subcutaneously implanted pacemaker. J Thorac Cardiovas Surg 1961; 814-30
Patient 13 was the first child to be operated on by the Buffalo group. The author (Stafford I Cohen) was unable to learn the exact dates of this child's operations after direct correspondence with Wilson Greatbatch, a search of Buffalo, New York, newspapers and contact with the librarian/archivist at the Children's Hospital of Buffalo, New York, where Dr. Norman B Thompson practiced and was stated to have treated this seven-year-old child in association with William Chardack and Wilson Greatbatch

15. Frank HA, Hurwitz A, Seligman AM. The treatment of hypoprothrombinemia with synthetic Vitamin K. N Engl J Med 1939; 221: 975

16. Frank HA, Fine J. Traumatic shock V. A study of the effect of oxygen on hemorrhagic shock. J Clin Invest 1943; 22: 305

17. Frank HA. Medical progress. Present-day concepts of shock. N Engl J Med 1953; 249: 445

18. Frank HA, Seligman AM, Fine J. Treatment of uremia after acute renal failure by peritoneal irrigation. JAMA 1946; 130: 703-05

19. Frank HA, Hall FM, Steer ML. Preoperative location of nonpalpable breast lesions demonstrated by mammography. N Engl J Med 1976; 295: 259-60

20. Frank HA, Zoll PM, Linenthal AJ. Surgical aspects of long-term electrical stimulation of the heart (eight-year experience). J Thorac Cardiovasc Surg 1969; 57: 17-30

21. Frank HA, Zoll PM. Surgical sepsis involving permanently implanted mechanical and electrical devices. Presented to the International Surgical Society. Moscow, USSR, August 1971

22. The boy with the electrical heart. Newsweek November 28, 1960: 80

23. Letter from Howard Frank to Samuel Schuster November 15, 1960. On file. With permission

24. Letter on file. With permission

25. Sells Furniture...The Daily Courier (Connellsville, PA) November 11,1961: 9

26. Gifts flood heart boy by admirers of pluck. Unknown Boston newspaper November 1960. Courtesy of Alan Belgard. With permission

27. Hospital tears up $2,484 bill for boy. Valley Independent (Morriser, PA) November 11, 1961 (UPI)

28. Cohen SI. Dr Benedict Massell. Profiles in cardiology. Clin Cardiol 32, 8, E68-E69 (2009) (www.interscience.Wiley.com) DOI: 10.1002/ clc 20536©2009 Wiley Periodicals Inc

29. Sells Furniture...The Daily Courier (Connellsville, Pa) November 11, 1961: 9

30. Harold Siddons and Edgar Sowton. Cardiac Pacemakers. Springfield, Illinois: Charles C Thomas Publisher, 1967; Table VI: 80-83

FIFTEEN

1. Lown B, Bey SK, Perloff MA, Abe T. Cardioversion of ectopic tachycardias. Am J Med Sci 1963. 246: 257-264 (presented at Atlantic City May 1, 1963)

2. Tom McNichol. AC/DC. The Savage Tale Of the First Standards War. San Francisco: Jossey-Bass. A Wiley Imprint, 2006

3. Man's heart stops, revived for 4 hours. New York Times; July 28, 1948: D7. The surgeon did not wish to be identified

4. The film is mentioned in Jude JR. Personal reminiscences of the origin and history of cardiopulmonary resuscitation (CPR). Am J Cardiol 2003; 92: 956-63

5. Philip Gold. Correspondence to Stafford I Cohen August 06, 2008. With permission

6. Hooker DR, Kouwenhoven WB, Longworthy OR. The effect of alternating current on the heart. Am J Physiol 1933; 103: 444-54. Herein lies the explanation of why house-circuit alternating current is more likely to cause, rather than terminate, ventricular fibrillation. High voltage AC shock of 150-750 volts was the range used by Zoll to be delivered during a brief duration. House circuits deliver 110 volts in the United States. Low voltage does not depolarize the entire heart. The parameters for Canadian house current in 1963 are unknown to the author

7. Harvey Sigman. Correspondence to Stafford I Cohen June 26, 2008. With permission

8. Barouh Berkovits interviewed by Stafford I Cohen October 30, 2009. With permission

9. Direct Current defibrillation had been successfully applied to closed-chest animals by Sanford Leeds, Arthur Guyton, Nuam Gurvich and William Kouwenhoven, among others

10. The letters in sequence follow:

   a. February 08, 1961. From Sidney Alexander to Barouh Berkovits requesting that information be sent to Dr. Lown about the principles of defibrillation and the characteristics of a good defibrillator

   b. February 17, 1961. From Sidney Alexander to Barouh Berkovits thanking Barouh for information and a request to test the capacitor discharge defibrillator under development

   c. April 10, 1961. From Bernard Lown to Barouh Berkovits. This letter is included in reference 11 below by Cakulev

   d. May 03, 1961. The last of the series after the delivery of the defibrillator. The letters were supplied by Barouh Berkovits during interview by Stafford I Cohen October 30, 2009, and by Sidney Alexander during an interview by Stafford I Cohen April 24, 2011. With permission

11. The letter dated April 10, 1961 was referenced in Cakulev I, Efimov, Waldo A. Cardioversion. Past, present and future. Circulation 2009; 120: 1623-32. Bernard Lown formally asked permission to test the Berkovits defibrillator

12. Lown B, Neuman J, Amarasingham R, Berkovits B. Comparison of alternating current with direct current electroshock across the closed chest. Am J Cardiol 1962; 10: 223-33

13. Wiggers CJ, Wégria R. Ventricular fibrillation due to single, localized induction and condenser shocks applied during the vulnerable phase of ventricular systole. Am J Physiol 1940; 128: 500-05

14. Barouh Berkovits interviewed by Stafford I Cohen February 15, 2010. With permission

15. Sidney Alexander interviewed by Stafford I Cohen April 24, 2011. With permission

16. Barouh Berkovits interviewed...February 15, 2010. With permission

17. Ruppel ES. The heart saver. Technol Rev 1982; June-July: 43-52

18. Lown B, Amarasingham R, Newman J, Berkovits B. The use of synchronized direct current countershock in the treatment of cardiac arrhythmias. J Clin Invest 1962; 41: 1381 (Abstract)

19. Sidney Alexander interviewed by Stafford I Cohen April 24, 2011. With permission

20. Bernard Kosowsky interviewed by Seymour Furman March 18, 2001. With permission to reference the selected content from the NASPE/HEART RHYTHM SOCIETY Rhythm in Time interviews

21. Albert Hyman interviewed by Stafford I Cohen October 28, 2011. With permission (No relation to Albert Hyman who invented the Hymanotor)

22. Ibid

23. Paul Axelrod interviewed by Stafford I Cohen October 01, 2009. With permission

24. Conference on artificial pacemakers and cardiac prosthesis. Sponsored by The Medical Electronics Center of the Rockefeller Institute, 1958. Jeffrey K, ed. PACE; 16: 1445-82. An unedited version of the conference contains the chairman's remarks. It is on file with Stafford I Cohen

25. Zoll PM. The intermediate history of cardiac pacing. In Harthorn JW, Thalen HJTh, eds.The Hague- The Netherlands: Martinas Nighoff Medical Division, 1973: 31

26. David KC Cooper, MD. Open Heart. The Radical Surgeons Who Revolutionized Medicine. New York: Kaplan Publishing, 2010: 78

27. Lefamine AA, Amarsingham R, Harkin D, Berkovits B, Lown B. A comparison of direct-current and alternating current defibrillation, under conditions of hypothermia. J Clin Invest 1962; 41: 1378-9 (abstract)

28. Zoll PM, Linenthal A. AC and DC countershock for arrhythmias. Letter to the editor. JAMA 1964; 188: 255

29. Zoll PM. Electric Countershock for Cardiac arrhythmias. Isr J Med Sci 1967; 3(2): 313-17.The author (Stafford I Cohen) witnessed one of the five episodes of elective AC conversion that resulted in ventricular fibrillation. After normal rhythm was restored with an immediate second countershock, a medical student asked Paul Zoll "Does that happen all the time?" Zoll's mono-word answer was, "No." When the student departed Zoll muttered, "He doesn't know much."

30. Zoll PM. Development of electrical control of cardiac rhythm. JAMA 1973; 226: 881-86

31. Zoll PM. A history of electrical cardiac stimulation. In Thalen HJTh. ed. Cardiac Pacing. The Netherlands: Van Gorcum & Comp BS Assen, 1973: 8

32. Lown B, Perlroth MG, Kaidbey S, Abe T, Harken D. "Cardioversion" of atrial fibrillation. N Engl J Med 1963; 269: 325-31

33. Paul Axelrod interviewed ... October 01, 2009. With permisson

34. Milton Paul interviewed by Stafford I Cohen November 16, 2001. With permission

35. Paul MH, Miller RA. External electric termination of supraventricular arrhythmias in congenital heart disease. Circulation 1962; 25: 604-09

36. Zoll PM, Linenthal AJ. Termination of refractory tachycardia by external countershock. Circulation 1962; 25: 596-603

37. Milton Paul interviewed ... November 16, 2001. With permission

38. Paul Minton interviewed by Stafford I Cohen July 28, 2008. With permission

39. Ross Zoll. Correspondence to Stafford I Cohen August 02, 2006. With permission

40. Ross Zoll interviewed by Stafford I Cohen February 09, 2009. With permission

41. Pantridge JF, Geddes JS. A mobile intensive care unit in the management of myocardial infarction. Lancet 1967; 2: 271-73

42. Pantridge JF. Mobile coronary care. Chest,1970; 58: 229-34

43. Mirowski M, Mower MM, Staewen WS, Tabatznik B, Mendeloff AI. Standby automatic defibrillator. Arch Int Med 1970; 126: 159-61

44. Mirowski M, Mower MM, Staewen WS, Denniston RH, Tabatznik B, Mendeloff AI. Ventricular defibrillation through a singular intra-vascular electrode system. Clin Res 1971; 19: 328 (abstract)

45. Mirowski M, Mower MM, Langer A, Heillman MS, Schreibman J. A chronically implanted system for automatic defibrillation in active conscious dogs: experimental model for treatment of sudden death from ventricular fibrillation. Circulation 1978; 58: 90-4

46. Mirowski M, Reid PR, Mower MM, Watkins L, Gott VL, Schauble JF, Langer A, Hellman MS, Kolenik SA, Fischell RE, Weisenfeldt ML. Termination of malignant

ventricular arrhythmias with an implanted automatic defibrillator in human beings. N Engl J Med 1980; 303: 322-24

47. Paul Axelrod interviewed … October 01, 2009. With permission

48. Lown B, Axelrod P. Implanted standby defibrillators. (Editorial) Circulation 1972; XLVI: 637-39

49. Kastor JA. Michel Mirowski and the automatic implantable defibrillator. Am J Cardiol 1989; 63: 1121-6

50. Paul Zoll in discussion with Stafford I Cohen. Personal observation without recollection of date

51. Barouh Berkovits interviewed… October 30, 2009. With permission

SIXTEEN

1. Alexander Pope. An Essay On Criticism (71).Pt 1: 1-135

2. Ross Zoll interviewed by Stafford I Cohen February 09, 2009. With permission

3. Ibid

4. Ross Zoll. Correspondence to Stafford I Cohen August 02, 2006. With permission

5. Alan Belgard interviewed by Stafford I Cohen March 10, 2012. With permission

6. Panel discussion – II. C Walton Lillehei chairman. In Cardiac Pacemakers. Ann NY Acad Sci 1964; 111: 955

7. Conference on artificial pacemakers and cardiac prosthesis. Sponsored by the Medical Electronics Center of the Rockefeller Institute, 1958. Jeffrey K, ed. PACE 1993; 16: 1445-82

8. Cardiac Pacing and Cardioversion. Meltzer LE, Kitchell JR, eds. Philadelphia: The Charles Press, 1967: 75

9. Wilson Greatbatch. The Making Of The Pacemaker. Amherst, New York: Prometheus Books, 2000: 52

10. Bernard Kosowski interviewed by Seymour Furman March 10, 2001. With permission to reference the selected content from the NASPE/ HEART RHYTHM SOCIETY Rhythm in Time interviews

11. Stafford I Cohen. Temporary and permanent pacemakers. In Cardiac Catheterization Angiography and Intervention. Fourth Edition. Grossman W, Baim D, eds. Philadelphia, London: Lea & Febiger, 1991: 396-418

12. Zoll RH, Zoll PM, Frank HA, Belgard AH. A new self-retaining myocardial electrode. Cardiac Pacing. Pacemaker Technology. Presented at the Second European Symposium on Cardiac Pacing 1981. Padova Italy: Piccin Medical Books, 1982: 1125-28

13. Ott DA, Gillette PC, Cooley DA. Atrial pacing via the subxyphoid approach. Tex Heart Inst J 1982; 9(2): 149-52

14. Dunn JM, Mehta AV. Cardiac pacing in children. In Ideal Cardiac Pacing. Hakki A-H, ed. In the series Major Problems in Clinical Surgery. W.B. Saunders Company, 1984: 120-26

15. Panel discussion. William WL Glenn moderator. Advances in Cardiac Pacemakers. Seymour Furman consulting ed. Ann NY Acad Sci 1969; 167: 622-26

16. Zoll PM, Linenthal AJ, Norman LR. External electrical stimulation of the heart in cardiac arrest. Arch Int Med 1955; 96: 639-53

17. Zoll PM, Linenthal AJ, Gibson W, Paul MH, Norman LR. Intravenous drug therapy of Stokes-Adams disease. Circulation 1958; 17: 325-39

18. Linenthal AJ, Zoll PM. Prevention of ventricular irritability in Stokes-Adams disease by intravenous sympathomimetic amines. Circulation 1963; 27: 1-4

19. Zoll PM. Drug therapy and external pacing. Ann NY Acad Sci 1969; 167: 576-81

20. Zoll PM, Zoll RH, Belgard AH. External noninvasive electrical stimulation of the heart. Crit Care Med 1981; 9: 393-94

21. Paul Zoll interviewed by Kirk Jeffrey February 05, 1990. With permission to reference the selected content from the NASPE/HEART RHYTHM SOCIETY Rhythm in Time interviews.

22. Ross Zoll interviewed … February 09, 2009. With permission

23. Condorelli L. Tentativo di terapia in syndrome di Adams-Stokes. Ritmo ventricolare artificialment mantinuto per due ore mediante stimolazioni meccaniche. Minerva Med 1928; 8: 343-50

24. Link MS, Maron BJ, Wang PJ, VanderBrink VA, Zhu W, Estes M. Upper and lower limits of vulnerability to sudden arrhythmic death with chest-wall impact (commotio cordis). JACC 2003; 41: 99-104

25. Lown B. The antiarrhythmic blow to the sternum: Thump version. Heart Rhythm 2009; 6(10): 1512-13. E pub 2009 August 22

26. Basic Research Is The Starting Point. A brochure published by The American Heart Association. Date uncertain: 13

27. Zoll PM, Belgard AH, Weintraub MJ, Frank HA. External mechanical cardiac stimulation. N Eng J Med 1976; 294: 1274-75

28. Cohn P, Angoff GH, Zoll PM, Sloss LJ, Markis J, Graboys T, Green L, Braunwald E. A new noninvasive technique for inducing post-extrasystolic potentiation during echocardiogram. Circulation 1977; 56: 598-605

29. Angoff GH, Wistran D, Sloss LJ, Markis J, Come P, Zoll PM, Cohn P. Value of noninvasively induced ventricular extrasystole during echocardiographic and phonocardiographic assessment of patients with idiopathic hypertrophic subaortic stenosis. Am J Cardiol 1978: 42: 919-23

30. Blatt CM, Lown B, Rabinovitz SH. A noninvasive means of assessing glycoside toxicity: mechanically induced repetitive ventricular response. Proc Soc Exp Biol Med 1977; 156: 531-33

31. Lown B, Verrier RL, Blatt CM. Precordial mechanical stimulation for exposing electrical instability in the ischemic heart. Am J Cardiol 1978; 42: 425-28

32. Ibid

SEVENTEEN

1. Mary Zoll interviewed by Stafford I Cohen July 26, 2011. With permission

2. Elliot Mahler interviewed by Stafford I Cohen September 19, 2007. With permission

3. Wilson Greatbatch. The Making of the Pacemaker. Amherst, New York: Prometheus Books, 2000: 33

4. Jeanne Rogers and family interviewed by Stafford I Cohen July 27, 2006. With permission

5. Ibid

6. Zoll PM. Development of electrical control of cardiac rhythm. JAMA 1973; 226: 881-86

7. Jeanne Rogers…interviewed by Stafford I Cohen July 27, 2006. With permission

8. Ibid

9. Ross Zoll interviewed by Stafford I Cohen February 9, 2009. With permission

10. Invitation on file

11. The Albert Lasker Medical Research Awards Program; 1973: 3

12. David Kaplan interviewed by Stafford I Cohen February 01, 2008. With permission

13. Merrill Cohen. Correspondence to Stafford I Cohen December 02, 2007. With permission. The letter from Paul Zoll to Merrill Cohen dated December 05, 1973 is on file

14. Frederica Sigel interviewed by Stafford I Cohen March 01, 2008. With permission

15. It is unclear why there was no further action or information about the status of the nomination. The papers might not have been submitted. The application might have been untimely because Paul Zoll was in the twilight of his career. It is unknown if this was the first, the last, or the only formal Nobel initiative

16. Albert Lasker Clinical Medical Research Awards. Citations. JAMA 1973; 226: 876

17. Harken DE. Pacemakers, past-makers, and the paced: an informal history from A to Z (Aldini to Zoll). Biomed Instrum Technol 1991 Jul-Aug; 25(4): 319

18. Carl Orecklin described the course of his Stokes-Adams disease during two interviews. Carl Orecklin interviewed by Stafford I Cohen March 13, 2000 and January 09, 2008. Both with permission

19. Houser RG. Here we go again-Another failure of post marketing device surveillance. N Eng J Med 2012; 366: 873. One manufacturer issued a recall of two models of internal defibrillators because of potential lead failure that might result in serious injury or death. Seventy nine thousand patients are at risk in the USA. A prior recall by another manufacturer involved 268,000 patients

20. Thomas M Burton. FDA in hot seat on safety. The Wall Street Journal April 10, 2012: B1. The author reports 33 deaths related to the recalled faulty leads cited in reference #19 above

21. Edward Giberti interviewed by Stafford I Cohen November 26, 2008. With permission

22. Harken DE. Pacemakers,past-makers...Biomed...25(4); 319

23. Jeanne Rogers...interviewed by Stafford I Cohen July 27, 2006. With permission

EIGHTEEN

1. Zoll PM. Transcutaneous cardiac pacing. In The Leading Edge: Cardiology. Zipes DP, ed. A Matrix Communications Inc Publication 1987; 1: 1-3,7-8,11-12

2. Paul Zoll interviewed by Kirk Jeffrey February 5, 1990. With permission to reference the selected content from the NASPE/HEART RHYTHM SOCIETY Rhythm in Time interviews

3. Zoll R. 50th Anniversary of defibrillation: Paul M. Zoll MD and the beginning of Zoll Medical Corporation. EP Lab Digest 2006: 14-16

4. Ibid

5. Ross Zoll interviewed by Stafford I Cohen February 29, 2009. With permission

6. Ibid

7. Ibid

8. Nuremberg Code (1947). http://en.wikipedia.org/wiki/Nuremberg_Code

9. Falk RH, Zoll PM, Zoll RH. Safety and efficacy of noninvasive pacing. A preliminary report. N Engl J Med 1983; 309: 1166-70

10. Edmund "Leigh" Stein interviewed by Stafford I Cohen June 5, 2008. With permission

11. Ibid

12. Ibid

13. Thomas Claflin interviewed by Stafford I Cohen October 4, 2011. With permission

14. Rodney Falk interviewed by Stafford I Cohen November 14, 2010. With permission

15. Falk RH, Zoll PM, Zoll RH. Safety and efficacy…N Engl J Med 1983; 309: 1166-70

16. Zoll PM, Zoll RH, Falk RH, Clinton JE, Eitel DR, Antman EM. External noninvasive temporary cardiac pacing: Clinical trials. Circulation 1985: 71: 937-44

17. Zoll PM. Noninvasive temporary cardiac pacing. Journal of Electrophysiology (Futura) 1987; 1: 156-61

18. Edmund "Leigh" Stein interviewed… June 05, 2008. With permission

19. Rolf Stutz during memorial service for Paul M Zoll February 23, 1999. Courtesy of the Ruth and David Freiman Archives at Beth Israel Deaconess Medical Center. With permission

20. Ibid

21. Document on file with Stafford I Cohen

22. Warren Manning interviewed by Stafford I Cohen May 23, 2012. With permission

EPILOGUE

1. Personal experience. Stafford I Cohen. Date not recorded

2. Elliot Mahler interviewed by Stafford I Cohen September 19, 2007. With permission

3. Kong MH, Fonarow GC, Peterson ED, Curtis AB, Hernandez A, Sanders GD, Thomas KL, Hayes DL, AL-Khatib SM. Systematic review of the incidence of sudden death in the United States. JACC 2011; 57: 792-93

4. Ross Zoll interviewed by Stafford I Cohen February 9, 2009. With permission

5. Conference of Artificial Pacemakers and Cardiac Prosthesis. Sponsored by The Medical Electronics Center of the Rockefeller Institute 1958. Kirk Jeffrey ed. PACE 1993; 16: 1445-82

6. Cardiac Pacing and Cardioversion. Meltzer LE, Kitchell JR, eds. Philadelphia: The Charles Press, 1967: 75

APPENDIX ONE

1. Kite C. An essay on the recovery of the apparent dead. London; C. Dilly 1778. In Alzaga AG, Varon J, Baskett P. Charles Kite: The Clinical Epidemiology of Sudden Cardiac Death and the Origin of the Early Defibrillator. In Resuscitation Greats. Baskett PJF, Baskett TE, eds. Clinical Press Ltd, Redland Green Farm, Redland Bristol 1356 7HF UK, 2007: 54-59

2. Ibid: 28

3. Eisenberg MS. Charles Kite's essay on the recovery of the apparent dead. The first scientific study of sudden death. Ann Emerg Med 1994; 23: 1049-53

4. Senning Ä. Cardiac pacing in retrospect. PACE 1983; 145: 733-39

5. Mond HG, Sloman JG, Edwards RH. The first pacemaker. PACE 1982; 5: 278-82

6. Lidwill MC. Cardiac disease in relation to anesthesia. In Transactions of the Third Session, Australian Medical Congress (British Medical Association) Sidney Australia: Sept.2-7, 1929: 160 (Cited in Ref #5 above)

7. Furman S, Szarka G, Layvand D. Reconstruction of Hyman's second pacemaker. PACE 2005; 28: 446-58

8. Furman S, Jeffrey K, Szarka G, The mysterious fate of Hyman's pacemaker. PACE 2001; 24: 1126-37

9. Ibid: 1137

10. Hyman AS, Resuscitation of the stopped heart by intracardiac therapy. Arch Int Med 1930; 46; 553-68

11. Hyman AS. Resuscitation of the stopped heart by intracardiac therapy. II Experimental use of artificial pacemaker. Arch Int Med 1932; 50: 283-305

12. Hyman AS, Resuscitation of the stopped heart by intracardiac therapy.III Further studies of the dying heart. American Therapeutic Society Transactions 1934: 102-04

13. Hyman AS. Resuscitation of the stopped heart by intracardiac therapy. IV Further use of the artificial pacemaker. United States Naval Bulletin 1935; 33: 205-14

14. Albert S Hyman and Aaron E Parsonnet. Applied Electrocardiography. New York: The MacMillan Co, 1929

15. Albert S Hyman and Aaron E Parsonnet. The Failing Heart of Middle Life. Philadelphia, PA: F.A. Davis Company, 1933

16. Physician invents self-starter for dead man's heart. Popular Science 1933 October 10: 25

17. David Charles Schechter. Exploring the Origins of Electrocardiac Stimulation. Minneapolis, MN: Medtronic Inc, 1983: 90

18. Furman S, Jeffrey K, Szarka G. Hyman's Pacemaker.http://www.hrsonline.org/ep-history/topics_indepth/topics/hymanpacemaker.asp. This web site has been discontinued. Copy on file with author

19. Hyman AS, Resuscitation of the stopped heart by intracardiac therapy. II Experimental use of artificial pacemaker. Arch Int Med 1932; 50: 283-305

20. Matteson L. Millionaire demanded and got 28 more hours of life after he died. Indiana Evening Gazette (Indiana, Pennsylvania) June 13,1933: 12

21. San Antonio Express (San Antonio, Texas) February 11,1936: 4

22. Schechter DC. Background of clinical electrostimulation. VI Precursor apparatus and events to the electrical treatment of complete heart block. NY State J Med 1972; 72: 953-61

23. Ibid

24. Schechter DC. Exploring the origins of electrocardiac stimulation…Medtronic Inc, 1983: 91

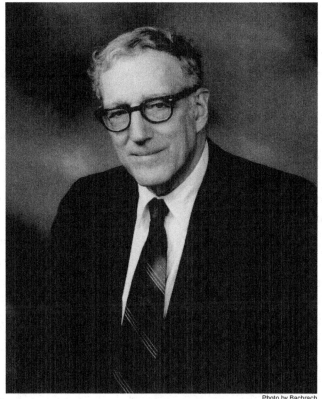

ABOUT THE AUTHOR

Stafford I. Cohen has been a licensed physician for 51 years. Before that, he graduated magna cum laude with a Bachelor of Arts degree from Brown University and pursued his medical training at the Boston University School of Medicine. He was a medical intern and a medical resident at Beth Israel Hospital, Boston. Licensed in internal medicine, Dr. Cohen became certified in cardiology after receiving sub-specialty training in the cardiology departments of Charles K. Friedberg at Mt. Sinai Hospital, New York, and Anthony Damato at the US Public Health Service Hospital, Staten Island, New York, where Dr. Cohen was a Research Associate. Dr. Cohen was a staff physician specializing in cardiology at Beth Israel Deaconess Medical Center, Boston, from 1968 to 2009. He continues to serve on the staff of Beth Israel

Deaconess. His current academic appointments are Associate Clinical Professor of Medicine at Beth Israel Deaconess Medical Center and Harvard Medical School.

Dr. Cohen is currently a fellow of the American College of Physicians, American College of Cardiology, and the American Heart Association. He is a member of the Heart Rhythm Society.

Awards and honors presented to Dr. Cohen include honorary membership in the Harvard Medical Alumni Association, and nominations for the S. Robert Stone Award for Teaching at Beth Israel Hospital and the Daniel D. Federman Outstanding Clinical Educator Award of Harvard Medical School. He was a recipient of the Women's Aid in Heart Research Award and is on the faculty of the Oliver Wendell Holmes Society of Harvard Medical School.

Stafford Cohen was born in Boston. He married Deborah Rosen. Together they have two children and four grandchildren.

Through his long career, Dr. Cohen has authored and co-authored many articles, research studies and similar papers, published in peer-reviewed medical and scientific journals, as book chapters, and elsewhere. *Paul Zoll MD, The Pioneer Whose Discoveries Prevent Sudden Death* is his first full-length book.

Dr. Cohen was a medical resident under Dr. Zoll and, later, a colleague at Beth Israel Hospital. His respect and admiration for Dr. Zoll created the impetus for writing the book. While some of the biographical material presented in its pages comes from the author's experiences and interactions with Zoll, the majority of information conveyed in the book was drawn from Cohen's seven years of research. That research included original interviews with many of Zoll's colleagues, some of his contemporary pioneers, patients and family members. It entailed extensive examinations of archival material encompassing professional articles published by Dr. Zoll and other articles from medical journals, newspapers and magazines, books on modern cardiac care, books about pioneers with similar interests, transcripts of third-party interviews, and additional sources.

For more information, or to contact Dr. Cohen, please visit staffordcohenmd.com.

INDEX

193

CPSIA information can be obtained
at www.ICGtesting.com
Printed in the USA
FSOW03n1227041116